# *Jasmine's*

# TAMIL KITCHEN

## ALOYSIUS ASEERVATHAM

This is a work of nonfiction.

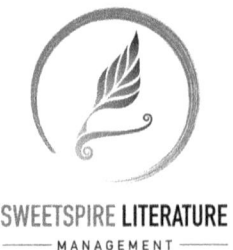

SWEETSPIRE LITERATURE
——— MANAGEMENT ———

# TABLE OF CONTENTS

100 RECIPES FROM

# *Jasmine's*
# TAMIL
# KITCHEN

# PREFACE

I grew up in a time and a place where men were not allowed in the kitchen. Instead, my four sisters learned to cook from our mother and grandmother and became experts. I must admit, I did not fight hard against that aspect of our culture! DI was a fussy eater during my early childhood and my mother made many varieties of food to get me to eat. By the time I was a young adult, I was fortunate to have experienced Sri Lankan Tamil cuisine in its entirety, courtesy of the talented women of my family - without ever having to spend time in the kitchen.

I married young, and my wife Jasmine, who at first could not cook like the women in my family but made it her mission to rival those around her, meticulously taking notes from talented cooks and eventually replicating delicious dishes. Our three sons had voracious appetites, and as we travelled around the world, she experimented with many varieties of food to keep pace with their changing tastes, exploring the depths of Sri Lankan Tamil cuisine. Consequently, I was a happy man with a happy belly and still a stranger to the kitchen!

When Jasmine was diagnosed with a terminal illness later in life, she began teaching me the basics of cooking so that I could look after myself after she passed away. In the short periods between her extended stays in the hospital, she took me on one joyful last journey through our kitchen. I learnt enough with her to become functional in the kitchen. I developed a keen interest in the art of cooking and borrowed recipes from my sisters and Jasmine's friends. If I am to believe my sons, I am now adept at making a large variety of Sri Lankan Tamil dishes, but I only know that I can cook the dishes I like and, more importantly, I enjoy eating them!

It took nearly a decade since my wife died before I truly appreciated the artistry that enabled my mother, sisters and wife to produce culinary delights. I cannot compare with their talents, so I have engaged my sisters and many of Jasmine's friends to help me compile this book. It is written for people who, like I began, are novices. The dishes are measured for two - for singles and couples who deserve the opportunity to experience the delight of cooking exotic, tasty food.

The Sri Lankan ladies who befriended Jasmine over the years, who shared recipes with her and who – on many occasions – hosted us and fed us with their Sri Lankan feasts have shared their unique recipes in Jasmine's memory. Together with some of Jasmine's favourites, they make up a selection of Sri Lankan Tamil dishes that will delight you and your kitchen.

*Aloysius Aseervatham*

*13 February 2024*

# ACKNOWLEDGEMENT

Twenty ladies helped me with the recipes in this book. I won't write about every one of them here, but I will single out three for special thanks.

Vasuki Sivananthan of Brisbane, Australia, inspired me when I first thought of compiling this recipe book. She felt that many people would benefit from a book of this kind: Sri Lankan children learning some Tamil cooking, single men and women experimenting with ethnic cuisine, couples with a taste for adventure and spice in the kitchen, and families seeking a variety of homely meals. She enthusiastically suggested some recipes of her own.

Pauline Samathar, near Birmingham in England, has my heartfelt thanks for expending a great deal of time and effort to provide me with several authentic recipes. Her wizardry in cooking is often referred to with awe by many Sri Lankan ladies.

Joyce Ferdinand, from Essex in England – a Chemical Engineer with expertise in food technology - not only supplied some of her own marvellous recipes but also worked tirelessly to structure this book so that the delights of Sri Lankan Tamil cuisine are more accessible to almost any cook.

I thank my sons Raj and Ratna for their advice on this book and their efforts to make it appealing to those of their generation and younger!

And Chandra Perera of Brisbane, thank you for your readiness to help me with the formatting of this book whenever I asked for it!

# THE CHEMICAL MELODY
# OF COOKING

Cooking is, at its very heart, a series of chemical reactions inspired by heat to create a symphony of taste.

The building blocks of your chemical reactions are your ingredients – your produce and your spices. They are your keys and your chords. Like a musical masterpiece, the combinations of these ingredients and the order in which you introduce these ingredients to each other and to the heat are all-important.

Of course, good music, however exquisite in composition, depends on the listener. We all have different taste buds, and what appeals to you may not appeal to someone else.

Remember, too, that not all keys and chords make good music. Some combinations and some sequences are terrible! So, too, in cooking, it is possible to make food you cannot stand eating, no matter what your taste buds are like.

A word of warning – unlike music, cooking carelessly can be harmful to your health! Meat, poultry and other foods can harbour dangerous micro-organisms. In Sri Lankan cuisine, as with many different cuisines, cooking meats to the correct temperature and for long enough is vital. Remember, in the kitchen, with great power comes great responsibility!

But the most important thing is to enjoy what you do in the kitchen. Enjoy your creativity, creations, and the joy they bring to you, your friends and your family. You will create memories for all your senses through the magic of your cooking.

.

# STRUCTURE OF THIS BOOK

This book is structured as follows:

1. Breakfast Options
2. Rice Dishes
3. Vegetable Dishes
4. Poultry and Egg Dishes
5. Beef, Lamb and Pork Dishes
6. Seafood Dishes
7. Pickles and Sambols
8. Salads
9. Soups
10. Snacks
11. Sweets and Desserts

Each recipe has been given a graded classification (Easy, Moderate and Challenging).

The recipes in this book have been chosen to fulfil two objectives: first and most importantly, they are proven versions of home-style Tamil recipes. Secondly, they can be accomplished by everyone, from the novice to the expert cook, who can modify and enhance the recipe as desired.

# SRI LANKAN
# TAMIL COOKING

Sri Lankan Tamil cooking has some influence from India, especially Kerala. Rice is usually consumed daily. It is eaten with spicy side curry dishes of vegetables, egg, meat, or seafood such as fish, squid, crab and prawns. This rice and curry meal is traditionally eaten at midday and often for dinner.

Sri Lankan Tamils are fond of Hoppers, String Hoppers, Pittu and Roti, which are made from rice flour and pancakes made from Urud Dhal Flour. These are eaten mainly for breakfast or dinner.

Other side dishes include pickles, chutneys and sambols, which can sometimes be very hot. The most famous of these is the coconut sambol, made of scraped coconut mixed with chilli peppers, dried Maldivian fish and lime juice.

A variety of snacks, tea and other beverages are consumed throughout the day. Yoghurt made from cow's milk and sago pudding (payasam) are served as dessert.

Eating outside of the home, although not common in the old days, has now become popular, especially among the wealthy and in the fast-paced society where both parents have to deal with a demanding work schedule.

There is some ethnic variation in food consumption. For instance, Muslims avoid pork, while Hindus avoid beef or are entirely vegetarians.

# SPICES
# AND
# CONDIMENTS

Spices and condiments are liberally used in dishes, and typically, people do not follow an exact recipe. Thus, every cook's curry will taste slightly different. Furthermore, people from different regions of Sri Lanka (for instance, hill-country dwellers versus coastal dwellers) traditionally cook in different ways. It is generally accepted for tourists to request that the food be cooked with a lower chilli content to cater for the more sensitive Western palate. Food cooked for public occasions typically uses less chilli than food cooked in the home.

Basic spices and condiments (in alphabetical order) for the kitchen include the following:

- **Asafoetida** is a taste enhancer and possesses medicinal properties.
- **Black Pepper** gives a spicy taste, and healing properties.
- **Cardamom** is used to garnish desserts.
- **Cinnamon** is a prominent spice because of its healing properties.

- **Clove** is strong and spicy.

- **Coriander** is used to garnish a dish.

- **Cumin** has a strong smell and taste.

- **Curry** leaves add flavour to curries.

- **Fennel seeds** have a strong aroma and flavour.

- **Fenugreek** has excellent healing properties.

- **Five spice powder** is a commonly used Chinese product.

- **Garlic** has many health benefits.

- **Ginger** has a spicy flavour and has healing properties.

- **Green and red chillies** are very spicy and add taste and smell.

- **Mustard** seeds have a good taste and aroma.

- **Tamarind** is alkaline, and so balances the taste of some of the spicy hot dishes.

- **Turmeric** adds a yellow colour and is a preservative.

# USEFUL EQUIPMENT FOR THE KITCHEN

- **A chopper** is used to chop onions and vegetables with ease.
- **Coconut scraper** is essential to scrape coconut if necessary.
- **A grinder** is handy to have to grind roasted or fried spices.
- **Measuring cups** of a standard size is a must in any kitchen.
- **Mortar and Pestle** are necessary for making curry paste or grinding various spices to make a mixture called garam masala.
- **A Rice Cooker makes cooking** rice easy.
- **Spice Rack** is helpful to have the essential spices in an easily accessible location.
- **The storage rack is good to have for the storage of spices that are** not used regularly.
- **A steamer is essential to have for steaming flour, vegetables,** etc.
- **String hopper mould and mats** are essential if making your own string hoppers.  String hoppers can be easily bought in restaurants.
- **Measuring scales**, whether traditional or digital, is a must in every kitchen, although many people use rough measurements after gaining some cooking experience.

# COMBINATION OF SPICES

Several combinations of spices are used to provide distinctive flavours to different dishes. It is better to prepare these in advance and keep them handy to use at the time of cooking. These can be bought from grocery shops.

## ROASTED CURRY POWDER FOR MEAT

Make your curry powder by mixing the following ingredients and roasting in low heat:

- Chilli powder; 2 tbsp.
- Coriander powder; 1 tbsp.
- Pepper powder; 1/2 tsp
- Cumin powder; 1 tsp
- Fennel powder; 1 tsp
- Spice powder; 1 tsp

**(Spice powder is made by mixing 1 tsp ground cinnamon, ½ tsp cardamom powder, 1/4 tsp crushed fennel seed, 1/4 tsp pepper (crushed) and 1/8 tsp ground cloves).**

# FISH CURRY POWDER

Make your fish curry powder by mixing the following ingredients:

- Raw chilli powder; 1 tbsp.
- Coriander powder; 1 tsp
- Fenugreek powder; 1 tsp.
- Black peppercorns; ½ tsp
- Sun dried chillies/ Paprika powder; 1 tbsp.
- Turmeric powder; ½ tsp
- Powdered ginger; 1 tsp
- Garlic powder; 1 tsp

# GARAM MASALA

Garam Masala is an aromatic blend of ground spices. Garam is a Hindi word meaning "Hot", and Masala means a "mixture of spices".

The mixture consists of cardamom, cloves and cinnamon. The proportion can vary according to one's taste. A suggested combination is one tablespoon of cardamom powder, one tablespoon of cloves and two cinnamon sticks of about 6 to 7 cm.

# *Jasmine's*
# TAMIL
# KITCHEN

## BREAKFAST OPTIONS

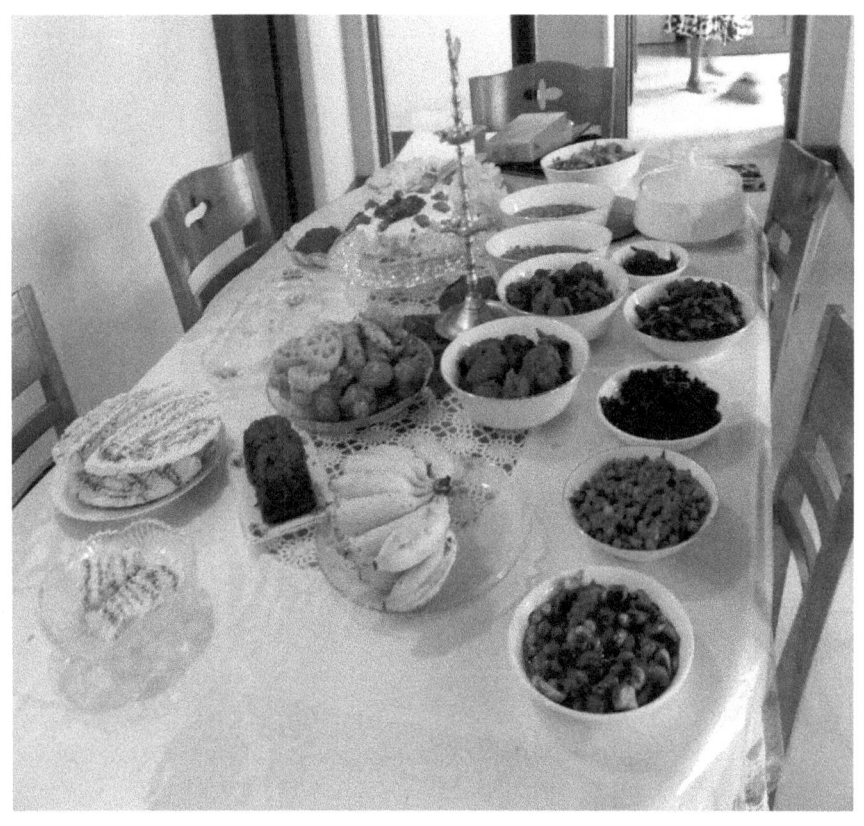

# Coconut Roti

## (EASY)

| INGREDIENTS |
| --- |

- **Plain flour (steamed);** 1 cup
- **Coconut (scraped);** 1/4 cup
- **Sugar;** 2 tbsp.
- **Water;** 1/2 cup or as needed
- **Salt;** to taste

## METHOD

1. Mix the flour, coconut, a little salt and sugar, and then add water and make a soft, sticky dough.

2. Warm a flat pan. Wet your fingers with water and take a lemon size ball of dough and put on the pan and press with the back of the wet fingers to make circles of roti of about 1 cm thick.

3. Cook both sides, till they turn golden brown.

# *Hoppers*

## (CHALLENGING)

| INGREDIENTS |
| --- |

- **Rice flour; (fine and raw)** 1 cup
- **Rice flour; (coarse and raw)** 1 cup
- **Bread mix flour; 1 cup**
- **Coconut milk powder;** 1/2 cup
- **Salt;** 1/2 tsp
- **Sugar;** 1/2 tsp
- **Water;** as required

## METHOD

1. Mix all the ingredients.
2. Add warm water and make a smooth paste (Hopper mix).
3. Keep overnight.
4. Make the hopper (called the plain hopper) in a very small frying pan by pouring the hopper mix (using a ladle) onto the centre of the pan, swirling it and cooking for a couple of minutes. Always cook with the lid on.

# NOTE:

Make **milk hoppers** by pouring 3 tbsp. coconut milk mixed with sugar onto the plain hopper while it is cooking.

Make **egg hoppers** in a similar manner by breaking an egg on to the plain hopper and cooking with lid on.

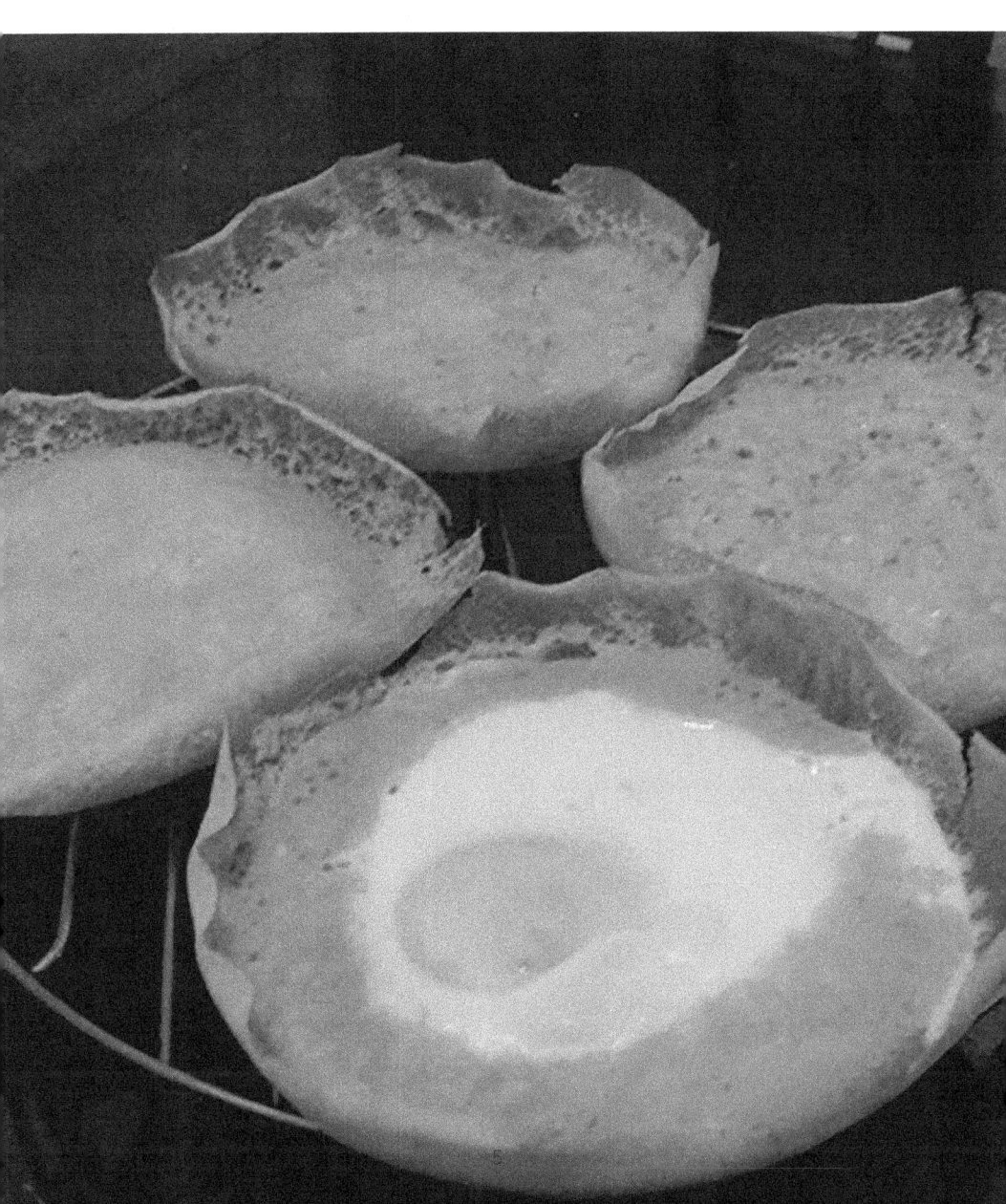

# *Idly*

## (CHALLENGING)

| INGREDIENTS |
| --- |
| • **Urud dhal;** 1 cup |
| • **Idly rice;** 2 cups |
| • **Yeast;** ½ tsp |
| • **Sugar;** ¼ tsp |
| • **Water;** as required |
| • **Salt;** to taste |

## PREPARATION

1. Soak the dhal and rice separately for at least 6 hours. Wash and drain.

2. Grind the dhal to a thick paste in a grinder/blender adding a little water.

3. Grind the rice to a slightly coarser texture adding a little water and into a thick paste.

4. Mix the yeast and sugar with 1 table spoon warm water in a cup and leave for few minutes to froth.

5.   Mix well the two pastes and the frothy yeast in a large bowl, add salt and allow to ferment for 8 hours or overnight.

## *METHOD*

1.   Stir the fermented mixture thoroughly.

2.   Lightly oil the Idly mould.

3.   Spoon in the paste and steam.

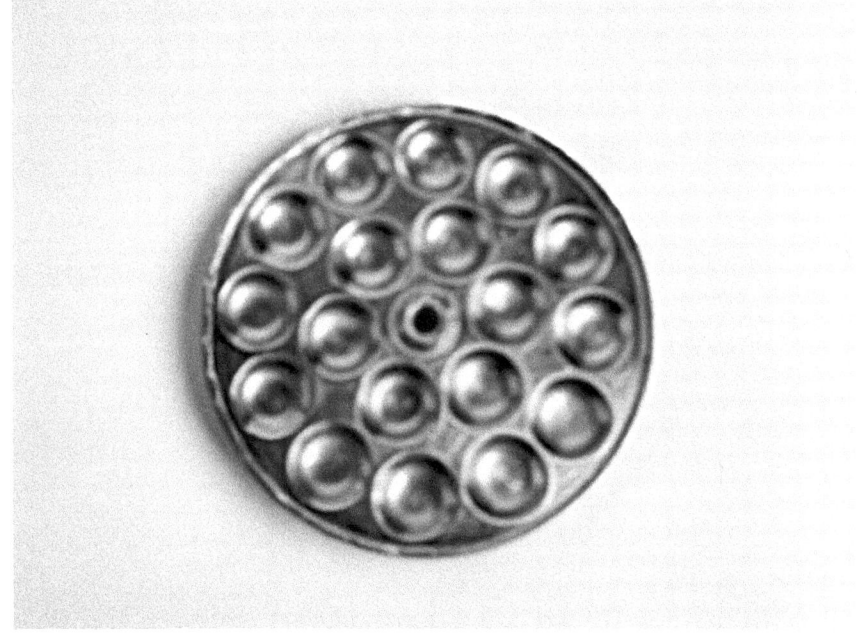

## VARIATION:

*Replace Idly rice with semolina.*

*Replace yeast and sugar with 1 tsp baking powder.*

# Kazhi (Kali)

## (EASY)

| INGREDIENTS |
| --- |

- **Red rice flour;** (roasted) 1/2 cup
- **Mung flour;** (roasted) 1/2 cup
- **Sugar;** 3 tbsp.
- **Coconut milk;** 1 cup
- **Water;** 1/2 cup
- **Salt;** to taste

## METHOD

1. Mix rice flour, mung flour, sugar and salt.
2. Add coconut milk and mix well.
3. Add water.
4. Cook on medium heat till the mixture thickens.

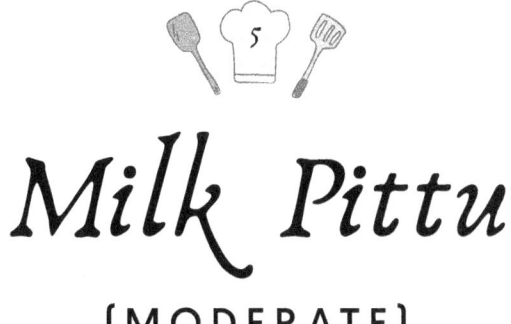

# Milk Pittu

## (MODERATE)

| INGREDIENTS |
| --- |
| • **Red rice flour; (roasted)** 1 cup |
| • **Mung flour; (roasted)** 1 cup |
| • **Water;** as needed |
| • **Coconut milk;** 1 tin |
| • **Sugar;** 5 tbsp. |
| • **Salt;** to taste |

## *METHOD*

1. Mix both flours and add salt to taste.

2. Make pittu by adding water little by little to the flour mixture and mixing with the back of a wooden spoon. (use an opened condensed milk tin to cut the big pieces of dough into small pieces)

3. Steam the pittu using a steamer and then transfer to a dish.

4. Heat the coconut milk and water and add sugar and salt. Keep 1 cup of this milk apart and mix the rest with pittu.

5. Ensure that the pittu and milk are not very hot to prevent the mixture becoming soggy.

6. Serve the pittu with the rest of the reserved milk.

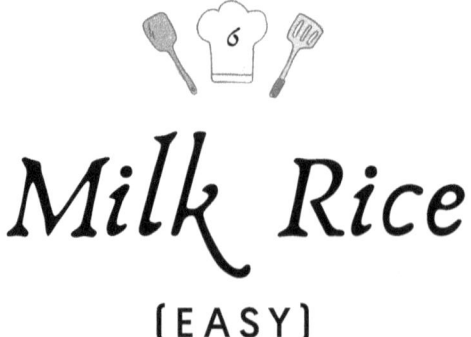

# Milk Rice

## (EASY)

| INGREDIENTS |
| --- |

- **Red raw rice;** 1 cup
- **Mung dhal (cleaned and roasted);** 2 tbsp.
- **Milk/ Coconut milk;** 2 cups
- **Sugar/Jaggery;** 4 tbsp.
- **Raisins;** 2 tbsp.
- **Cashew nuts (chopped);** 10
- **Cardamom;** 4 - 5
- **Water;** 1- 2 cups
- **Salt;** to taste

## *METHOD*

1. Wash the rice and mung dhal together and drain.
2. Cook the rice and dhal with water and 1 cup of milk and cardamom in a pan on medium heat.
3. Cook till the rice is soft adding more water if needed.
4. Add the remaining milk, cashew nuts, sugar, raisins and salt and heat till the mixture thickens.

# Milk Rice Porridge

## (EASY)

| INGREDIENTS |
|---|
| • **Red raw rice;** 1 cup |
| • **Water;** 4 ½ cups |
| • **Milk;** 1 cup |
| • **Coconut milk powder;** 2 tbsp. |
| • **Sugar;** 50 grams |
| • **Salt;** to taste |

## METHOD

1. Wash the rice and cook it with water and salt.

2. Add the milk, coconut milk powder and sugar and cook for another 10 minutes.

# Mumbai Toast

## (EASY)

### INGREDIENTS

- **Bread slices;** 3
- **Egg;** 1
- **Sugar;** 2 tsp
- **Vanilla;** 2 drops
- **Milk;** 1 cup
- **Butter/Margarine;** 1 tbsp.

## METHOD

1. Beat the egg.
2. Add sugar, vanilla and milk.
3. Soak the bread slice in the mixture.
4. Heat the butter/margarine in a non-stick pan.
5. Put the soaked bread one at a time in the pan, leaving it for one minute and then turning it and leaving for another minute (or until both sides become golden brown).

# Onion Roti

## (EASY)

| INGREDIENTS |
|---|
| • **Atta (or wheat) Flour;** 2 cups |
| • **Onions;** 2 |
| • **Green Chillies;** 4 small |
| • **Coconut (fresh or desiccated);** 1/4 cup |
| • **Water;** 1/2 cup |
| • **Sesame Oil;** 2 tbsp. |
| • **Salt;** to taste |

## *METHOD*

1. Mix the first four ingredients, add water and make a dough.

2. Add sesame oil, mix well, set aside in covered bowl for I hour.

3. Form several small balls, flattening each to desired thickness.

4. Fry (medium heat) on an oiled skillet turning roti until both sides are golden brown.

# Spicy Bread Toast

## (EASY)

| INGREDIENTS |
|---|
| • **Bread;** 2 slices |
| • **Eggs;** 2 |
| • **Green Chillies;** Half |
| • **Onion;** 1 small |
| • **Milk;** I tbsp. |
| • **Margarine;** 1 tbsp. |
| • **Pepper, ground;** 1 tsp |
| • **Salt;** to taste |

## *METHOD*

1. Make a paste using green chillies, onion and milk.

2. Beat the eggs with the paste, pepper and salt.

3. Soak the bread in the egg mixture .

4. Fry bread in margarine, turning the bread until both sides are golden brown.

# *String Hoppers*

## (CHALLENGING)

| INGREDIENTS |
| --- |
| • **Red rice flour (roasted); 1 cup** |
| • **White flour (steamed); 1 cup** |
| • **Boiled water; as required** |
| • **Salt; to taste** |

## METHOD

1.   Mix the red flour, white flour and salt in a bowl.

2.   Add the boiled water little at a time and make a soft dough to the right consistency to be able to make the string hoppers easily.

3.   Place small balls of the dough at a time in the string hopper press and press the top piston, making a circular motion, onto the string hopper mats thus creating the string hoppers.

4.   Boil some water in a reasonably large pan and place a steamer on top.

5.   Arrange four or five mats at a time in the steamer and close with a lid.

6. After steaming for about five minutes, take out the mats and tip the string hoppers off onto a plate.

7. Repeat the process till all the dough is used up.

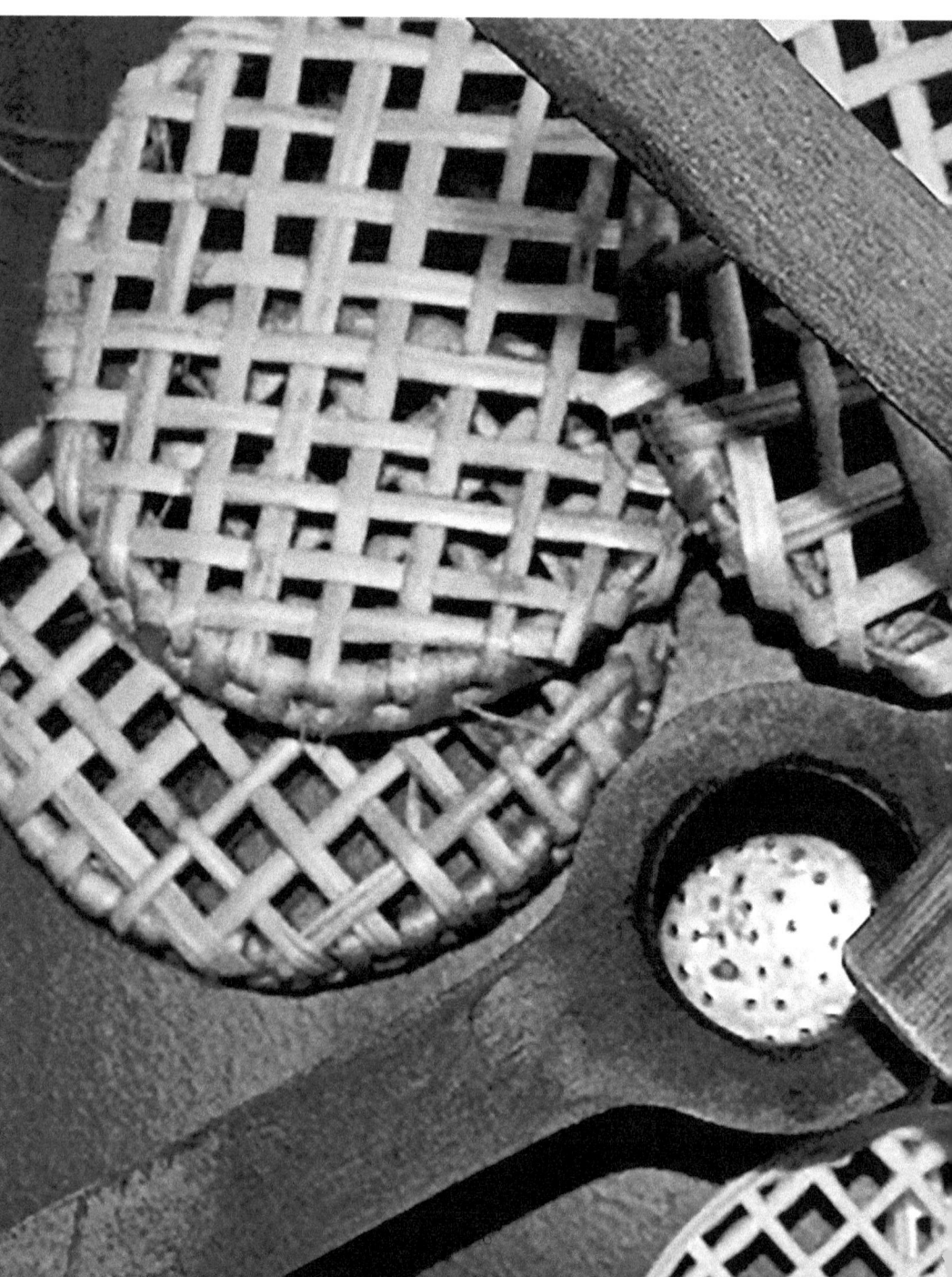

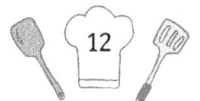

# Stuffed Pancake

## (CHALLENGING)

| INGREDIENTS |
|---|
| • **Self-raising flour;** 1 cup |
| • **Egg;** 1 |
| • **Milk;** 1 – 1 ½ cups |
| • **Yoghurt;** 2 tsp |
| • **Sugar;** 1 tsp |
| • **Salt;** to taste |

| INGREDIENTS FOR STUFFING |
|---|
| • **Fresh coconut;** 1/2 cup |
| • **Sugar;** 2 tbsp. |
| • **Cashew; (cut into small pieces)** – 25 grams |

## *METHOD*

1. In a bowl mix the self-raising flour, egg, yoghurt, salt and sugar and make a smooth batter by whisking with a hand beater, adding milk as required. Keep it aside for half an hour.

2. Roast the coconut (no need to add oil) in a frying pan adding the cashew half way.  When it turns golden brown add the sugar, mix well and roast for 2 minutes.  Keep it aside.

3. Using a ladle pour the batter onto the centre of the frying pan.

4. Immediately remove the frying pan from the heat and swirl it to form a pancake of a desired size and thickness.

5. Return the pan to the heat and when the surface of the pancake is not shiny turn it over using a spatula and cook the other side for a few seconds until very lightly browned. Spread 1- 1 ½ tbsp. of the coconut mixture on the pancake and roll it while hot.

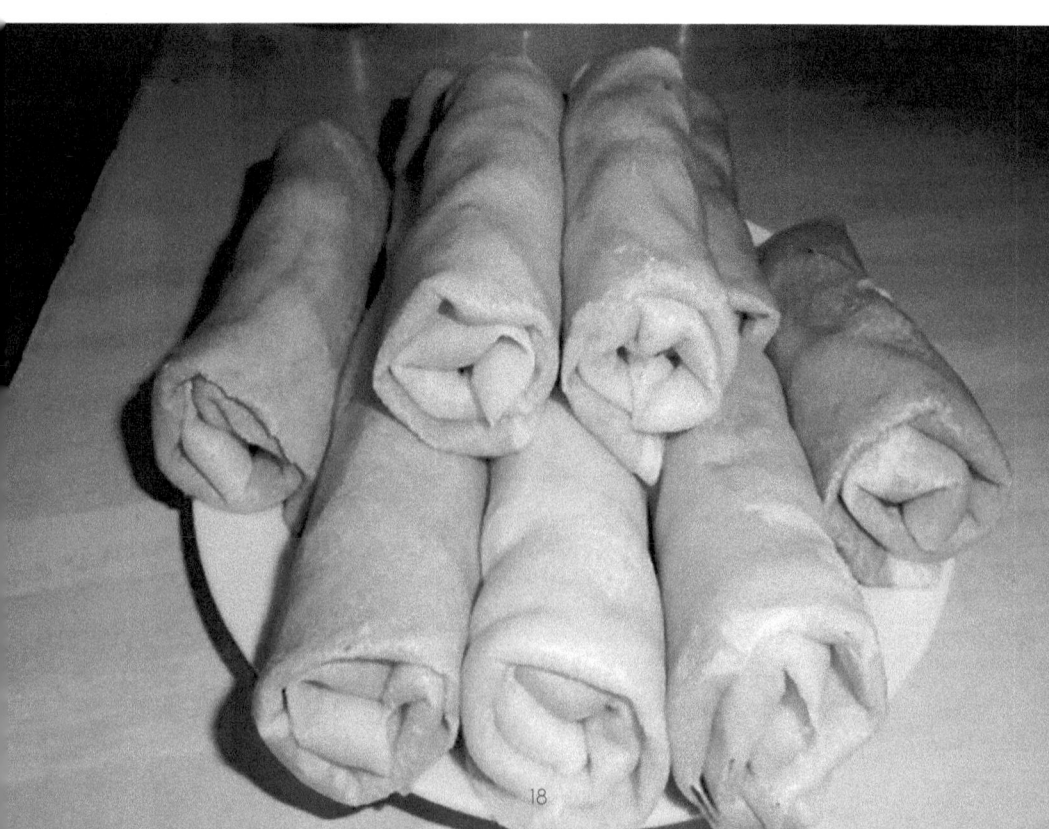

# Thosai

## (CHALLENGING)

### INGREDIENTS

- **Dhal (Urid);** 1 cup
- **Cooked rice;** 1/2 cup
- **Rice flour (white);** 1 cup
- **Onion (chopped);** 1
- **Fenugreek seeds;** 1 tbsp.
- **Gingili oil;** 2 tbsp.
- **Salt;** as required

## METHOD

1. Soak urid dhal and fenugreek in water separately for 4 to 5 hours.

2. Grind the urid dahl, fenugreek, cooked rice and chopped onions with sufficient water to get a fine paste.

3. After grinding add white rice flour and some more water (mix well) and keep overnight to ferment.

4. When the fermented thosai mixture is ready add salt.

5.   Now, temper the following in oil and add to the thosai mixture.

6.   Mustard seed; 1tsp    Onion (sliced); 1 small

7.   Cumin seeds; 1 tsp    Curry leaves; – 2 sprigs    Dry chilies; 2.

8.   Make the thosai on a non-stick skillet with little gingili oil spread on it

9.   Using a ladle, spread the thosai mix on the skillet, into a thin crepe.

10.  Let the thosai cook for 2-3 minutes and then turn and cook for another 1-2 min.

Note:   The thinner and crispier the thosai, the better it tastes.

# Uppuma

## (EASY)

| INGREDIENTS |
| --- |

- **Semolina;** 100 grams
- **Water;** 1 ½ - 2 cups
- **Red onions, sliced;** 1 or 2
- **Dry chillies, crushed;** 2
- **Mustard seed;** 1/2 tsp
- **Ginger, ground;** 1 tsp
- **Ghee (or butter);** 2 tbsp.
- **Curry leaves;** 1 sprig

## *METHOD*

1. Fry onions, chillies, curry leaves and mustard seed in 1 tbsp. ghee or butter.

2. Add semolina and stir to golden brown.

3. Add water to the mixture and keep stirring.

4. Add balance of the ghee or butter and stir for 5 minutes.

# *Jasmine's* TAMIL KITCHEN

## RICE DISHES

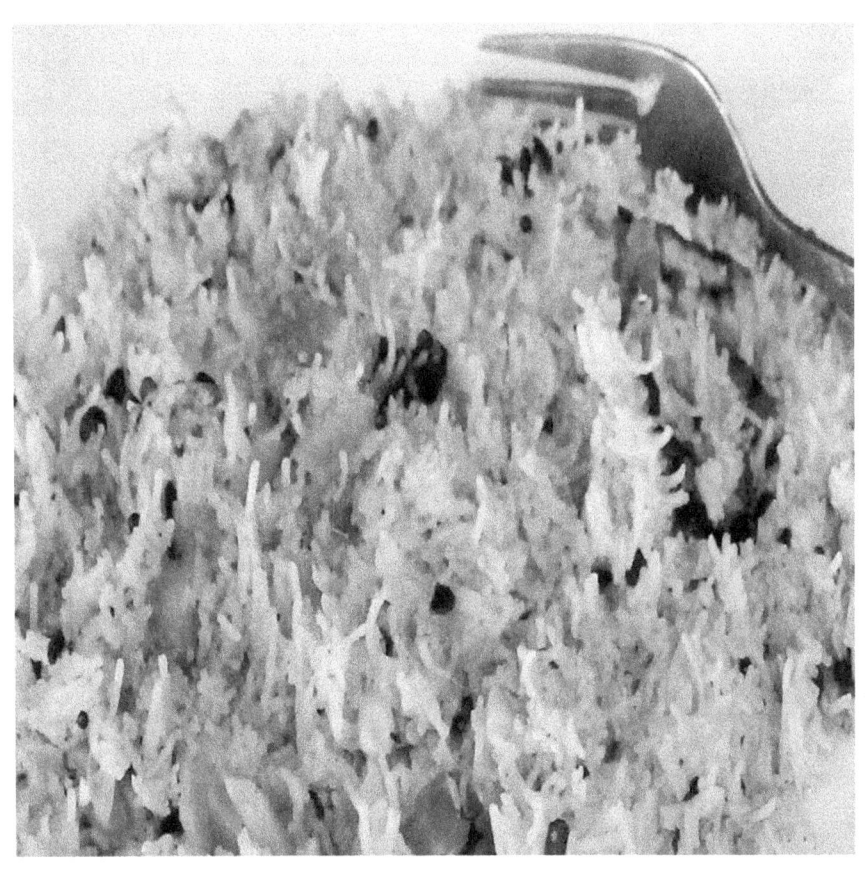

# METHODS OF COOKING RICE

## PAN METHOD

1.  Wash and drain 1 cup of rice.
2.  Add 2 cups of water and a little salt (optional).
3.  Bring to boil, stir and cover with lid.
4.  Turn the heat to "low "setting and cook for 12 – 15 minutes.
5.  Turn off heat and let it stand for 5 minutes.
6.  Fluff up the rice and serve.

## MICROWAVE METHOD

1.  Rinse and soak the rice in water for 30 minutes. Drain well.
2.  Place the rice in a deep microwaveable dish.
3.  Stir in twice the quantity of boiling water.
4.  Add salt and a teaspoon of butter or ghee (optional).
5.  Cover with cling film leaving a tiny vent on the side. Do not pierce the cling film.
6.  Cook on full power for 5 minutes.

7.  Turn the power to medium and cook for 10 minutes.

8.  Let the cooked rice stand for 5 minutes.

9.  Fluff up the rice and serve.

## RICE COOKER METHOD

1.  Place 1 cup of washed and drained rice in an electrically operated rice cooker.

2.  Add 2 cups of water and switch on.

    (When water is absorbed the cooker will turn itself off and will keep the rice warm).

# Coconut Rice

## (MODERATE)

| INGREDIENTS |
|---|
| • **Cooked rice;** 2 cups |
| • **Coconut milk;** 1 tin |
| • **Tempering ingredients** |
| • **Ghee or butter;** 1 tbsp. |
| • **Dried chillies (broken);** 2 |
| • **Mustard;** ½ tsp |
| • **Cumin seed;** ½ tsp. |
| • **Urud dhal;** 1 tbsp. |
| • **Ginger (chopped);** 1tsp |
| • **Green chilli (chopped);** 1 |
| • **Curry leaves;** few |
| • **Asafoetida;** ½ tsp |

## METHOD

1. Heat the ghee or butter in a frying pan and add mustard.

2. When the mustard seeds start to crackle add the dried chillies, cumin and urud dhal and stir.

3.   Add ginger, green chilli, asafoetida and curry leaves and saute until golden.

4.   Add coconut milk and the cooked rice and stir and cook until the milk is absorbed. Serve hot.

# *Curd Rice*

## (MODERATE)

### INGREDIENTS

- **Over cooked rice;** 2 cups
- **Thick yoghurt;** 1 ½ to 2 cups
- **Coriander (chopped);** 1 tbsp.
- **Salt;** 1 tsp

### TEMPERING INGREDIENTS:

- **Ghee or butter;** 1 tbsp.
- **Dried chillies (broken);** 2
- **Mustard;** ½ tsp
- **Cumin seed;** ½ tsp
- **Chana dhal;** 1 tbsp.
- **Urud dhal;** 1 tbsp.
- **Ginger (chopped);** 1tsp
- **Green chilli (chopped);** 1
- **Curry leaves;** few
- **Asafoetida;** ½ tsp

# METHOD

1. Combine the rice, alt, coriander and curd in a bowl and set aside.

2. Heat the ghee or butter in a frying pan and add mustard.

3. When the mustard seeds start to crackle add the dried chillies, Chana dhal and saute. (Chana dhal takes longer to cook than urud dhal).

4. Add cumin and urud dhal followed by ginger, green chilli, asafoetida and curry leaves. Saute until golden.

5. Pour the tempered ingredients onto the rice, stir and serve.

6. For richness mix a little cream.

# Dhal Rice

## (EASY)

| INGREDIENTS |
| --- |

- **Rice (any normal rice);** 1 cup
- **Dhal;** 1 cup
- **Onion;** 1.
- **Butter or ghee;** 1 tsp
- **Curry leaves;** 1 sprig
- **Dry chilli;** 1
- **Cardamom;** 2
- **Water;** (as needed)
- **Salt;** a pinch

## METHOD

1. Soak the dhal in water for 10 minutes.
2. Wash the rice.
3. Heat the butter, onion, chilli, curry leaves and cardamoms in a pan.
4. Add the rice and salt when the onion browns..
5. Add some water and bring the rice to boil.
6. Add the dhal half way through and wait till the dhal and rice are cooked.

# Flavoured Green Gram and Rice

## (CHALLENGING)

| INGREDIENTS |
| --- |

- **Rice (washed, soaked for 15 minutes);** 150 grams
- **Green grams (split grams);** 75 grams
- **Ghee;** 1 tbsp.
- **Water;** 1 ¼ cups
- **Onion (finely chopped);** 1
- **Garlic (crushed);** 1 clove
- **Ginger (shredded);** 1/2 a small piece
- **Green chillies (chopped);** 2
- **Cloves;** 2 whole
- **Cinnamon stick;** 1 piece
- **Green cardamoms;** 2 whole
- **Turmeric;** 1/2 tsp
- **Salt;** to taste

# METHOD

1. Gently heat the ghee in a medium heavy pan with a tight - fitting cover and fry the onion, garlic, ginger, chillies, cloves, cinnamon, cardamoms, turmeric and salt until the onion is soft and translucent.

2. Wash and drain the rice and gram; add to the spices and sauté for 2-3 mins. Add the water and bring to the boil. Reduce the heat, cover and cook for about 20-25mins or until all the water is absorbed.

3. Take the pan off the heat and leave to rest for 5 mins. Just before serving gently toss the mixture with a flat spatula.

# Fried Rice
# with Vegetables

## (MODERATE)

### INGREDIENTS

- **Rice;** 1 cup
- **Water;** 2 cups
- **Ghee or Butter;** 3 tbsp.
- **Ginger (crushed);** small piece
- **Garlic (crushed);** 2 cloves
- **Cinnamon;** small stick
- **Cardamom;** 5 pods
- **Turmeric;** ¼ tsp
- **Salt;** to taste

### *Vegetable Options*
*(one cup of any 2 or 3 vegetables sliced or chopped, from the following)*

**Leeks, Carrots, Mushroom, Peas, Spring Onion, Broccoli and Cauliflower.**

# METHOD

1.  Melt half of the ghee or butter in a pan

2.  Stir in ginger, garlic, cinnamon, cardamoms and turmeric.

3.  Add the rice and keep stirring until the rice is slightly fried. Add boiling water, cover and cook in medium to low heat for 15 minutes.

4.  Melt the rest of the Ghee or Butter in a wok. Add your preferred vegetables and stir fry.

5.  Mix in the cooked rice and serve.

# Mutton Biryani

## (CHALLENGING)

| INGREDIENTS |
| --- |

- **Mutton;** 200 grams
- **Rice (washed and drained);** 1 cup
- **Curd diluted with water;** 1/4 cup curd and 1 ½ cups water.
- **Ginger (pounded);** 1 small piece
- **Garlic (crushed);** 3 cloves
- **Onion (large);** 1
- **Mint leaves;** a few
- **Cardamom;** 2 or 3
- **Cinnamon (cut to pieces);** 1 small stick
- **Ghee or butter;** 2 tbsp.
- **Water;** 1 cup

# METHOD

1. Fry the onion in ghee or butter. Add the ginger, garlic, mint leaves, cardamom and cinnamon.

2. Add the rice and fry for a few more minutes.

3. Add the water and cook till the rice is three-quarter done and then remove from fire.

4. Make a dry mutton curry (refer to mutton curry recipe on page 148).

5. Take a big bowl and put a thin layer of rice and then a layer of mutton curry. Alternate the layer of rice and curry till the bowl is full.

6. Cover the bowl with aluminium foil and leave in in the oven at 200 degree Celsius for 20 minutes.

# Jasmine's
# TAMIL
# KITCHEN

## VEGETABLE DISHES

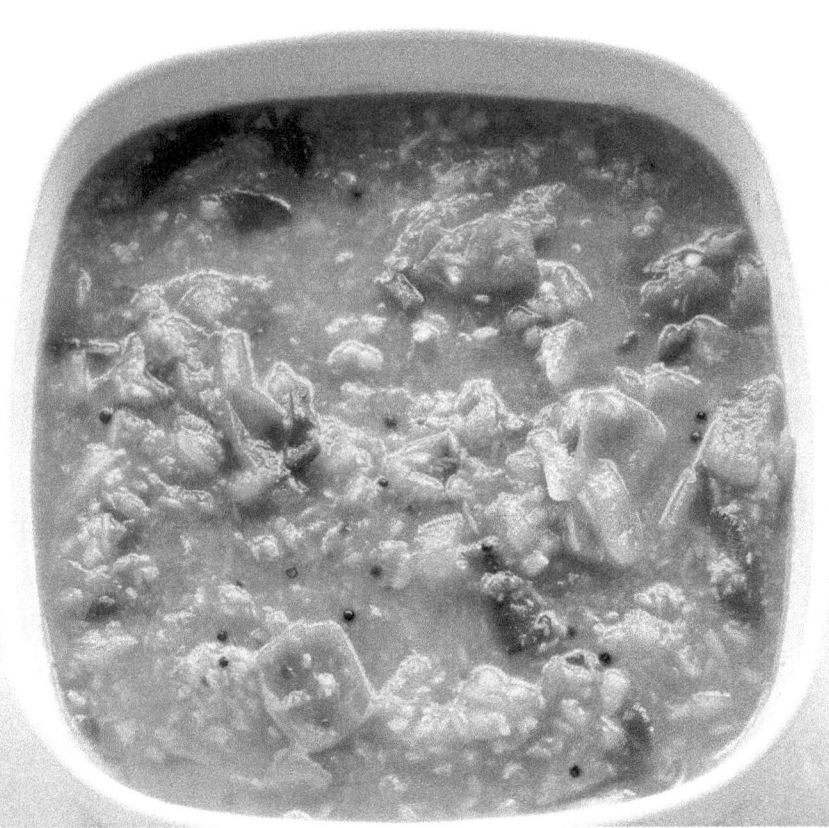

# Aubergine Milk Curry

## (MODERATE)

| INGREDIENTS |
|---|
| • **Aubergine (eggplant) (chopped);** 1 |
| • **Green chillies (sliced);** 2 |
| • **Onion (medium, chopped);** 1 |
| • **Oil;** 1tbsp. |
| • **Turmeric;** 1/2 tsp |
| • **Water;** 2 cups |
| • **Coconut milk;** 1/2 cup |
| • **Curry leaves;** 1 sprig |
| • **Lime or lemon juice;** 1 tsp |
| • **Salt;** to taste |

# METHOD

1. In a pan, sauté the onion in oil.

2. Add aubergine, green chillies, curry leaves, turmeric, salt and water. Stir, cover with lid and cook.

3. When water has reduced, add milk and cook for about 3 minutes stirring occasionally to stop aubergine sticking to the pan.

4. Add lime or lemon juice and serve.

**Note:** Cow's milk could be used instead of coconut milk and if preferred stir in a little single cream to enhance flavour and colour

# *Beans Curry*

## (MODERATE)

| INGREDIENTS |
|---|
| • **Green beans;** 200 grams |
| • **Oil;** 1 tbsp. |
| • **Onion (finely diced);** 1 |
| • **Garlic (sliced);** 2 cloves |
| • **Ginger (grated);** 1/2 tsp |
| • **Curry leaves;** 1 sprig |
| • **Chilli flakes;** 1 tsp |
| • **Cumin (powder);** 1/4 tsp |
| • **Turmeric powder;** 1/4 tsp |
| • **Coconut cream;** 1/4 cup |
| • **Maldives fish (dried, optional);** 1 tbs. |
| • **Salt;** to taste |

# METHOD

1.   Slice the end of the beans and cut into small pieces and Wash.

2.   Heat the oil in a pan or wok, stir fry the onions, garlic, and ginger and curry leaves for a few minutes.  Add beans and remaining ingredients and stir fry for a further 2 minutes.

3.   Add a little water and coconut cream. Simmer until the beans are tender.

4.   Add salt (to taste) and Maldives fish (if preferred).

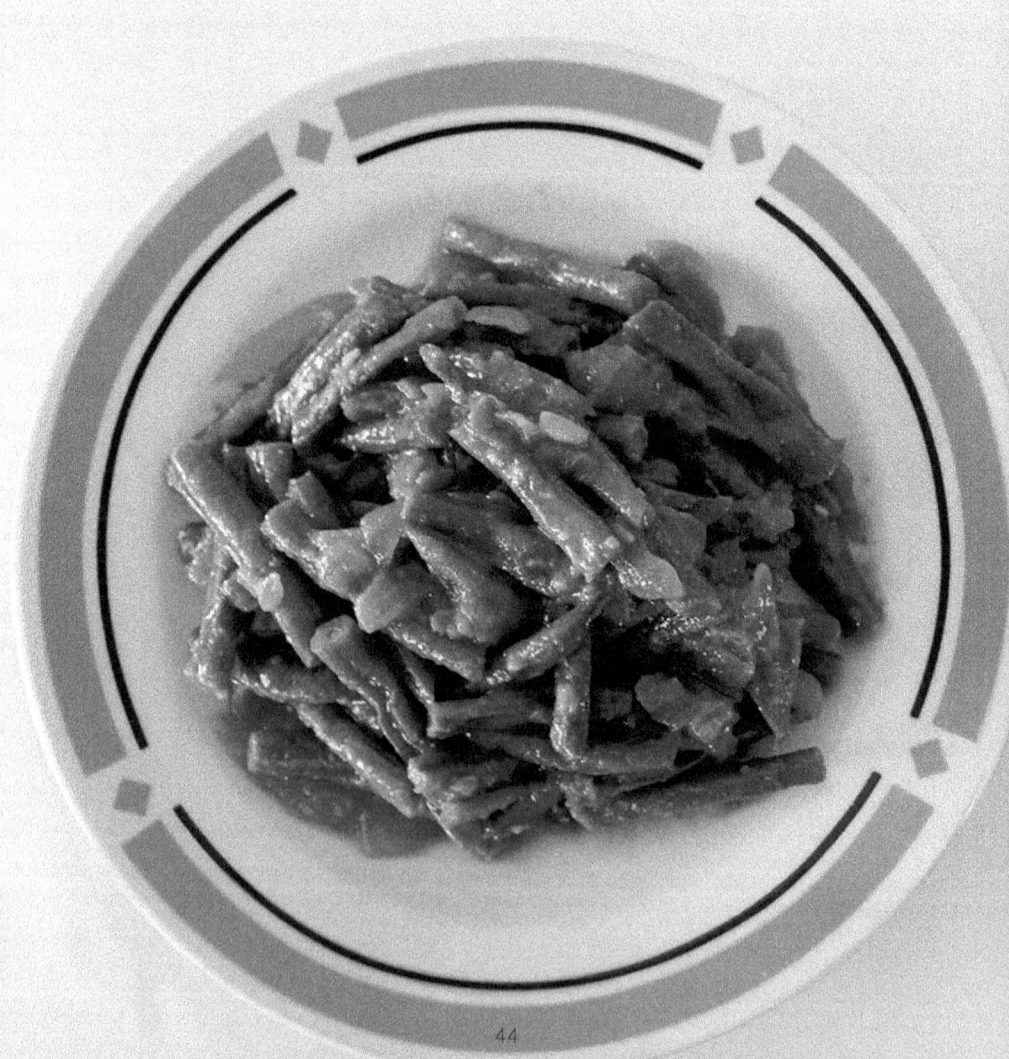

# Beetroot Curry

## (MODERATE)

| INGREDIENTS |
| --- |

- **Beetroot;** 500 grams
- **Oil;** 1 tbsp.
- **Mustard seeds;** 1/2 tsp
- **Fenugreek seeds;** 1/2 tsp
- **Curry leaves;** 1 sprig
- **Onion (finely chopped);** ½
- **Green chillies (slit);** 2
- **Chilli powder;** 1/4 tsp
- **Coconut milk;** 1/4 cup
- **Water; 1/2 cup
- **Salt and black pepper;** to taste

## METHOD

1. Peel the beetroot, wash and cut into small cubes and set aside.

2. Heat the oil and fry the mustard seeds and the fenugreek seeds.

3. When the mustard seeds begin to splutter, add the curry leaves, chopped onions and the green chillies and stir.

4.  Lower the temperature and add the chilli powder and stir quickly, so that the chilli does not get burnt.

5.  Add the beetroot and stir well and then add the salt and black pepper.

6.  Add the water, cover the pan with a lid and cook the beetroot for about 10 minutes.

7.  Once the beetroot is cooked add the coconut milk and cook for a further 10 minutes. Stir well and take the pan off the stove.

# Broccoli Stir-Fry

## (MODERATE)

| INGREDIENTS |
| --- |

- **Broccoli heads;** 250 grams
- **Onion (large, chopped);** 1
- **Green chillies (split);** 3
- **Garlic (chopped);** 2 pods
- **Desiccated coconut;** 1/4 cup
- **Saffron powder;** 1/4 tsp
- **Garam masala;** 1/2 tsp
- **Chilli powder;** 1/4 tsp
- **Fennel seeds;** 1/4 tsp
- **Mustard seeds (ground);** 1/4 tsp
- **Tuna fish;** small tin
- **Salt;** to taste

# METHOD

1. Shred the broccoli and cut the onion and green chillies into small pieces.

2. In a wok put the oil and fry the onion, green chillies, mustard seeds, fennel seeds and chopped garlic pods.

3. Mix the shredded broccoli, desiccated coconut, saffron powder, and chilli powder and garam masala.

4. When the broccoli looks cooked, empty a tin of tuna fish into this mixture and give it a stir.

# Cabbage and Carrot Stir-fry

## (MODERATE)

<table>
<tr><th>INGREDIENTS</th></tr>
</table>

- **Cabbage (shredded);** 50 grams
- **Carrots (grated);** 100 grams
- **Onion (small, chopped);** 1
- **Red chilli (broken into pieces);** 1
- **Mustard seeds;** 1/2 tsp
- **Cumin seeds;** 1/4 tsp
- **Curry leaves;** 1 sprig
- **Turmeric;** 1/4 tsp
- **Oil;** 2 tbsp.
- **Desiccated coconut;** 2 tbsp.
- **Chana dhal;** 1 tbsp.
- **Salt;** to taste

# METHOD

1. Fry the chopped onion, Chana dhal and red chillies in oil.

2. Add mustard seeds, cumin seeds & curry leaves.

3. Add carrots, cabbage, turmeric powder, and desiccated coconut.

4. Add salt and mix for about two minutes. Remove from stove.

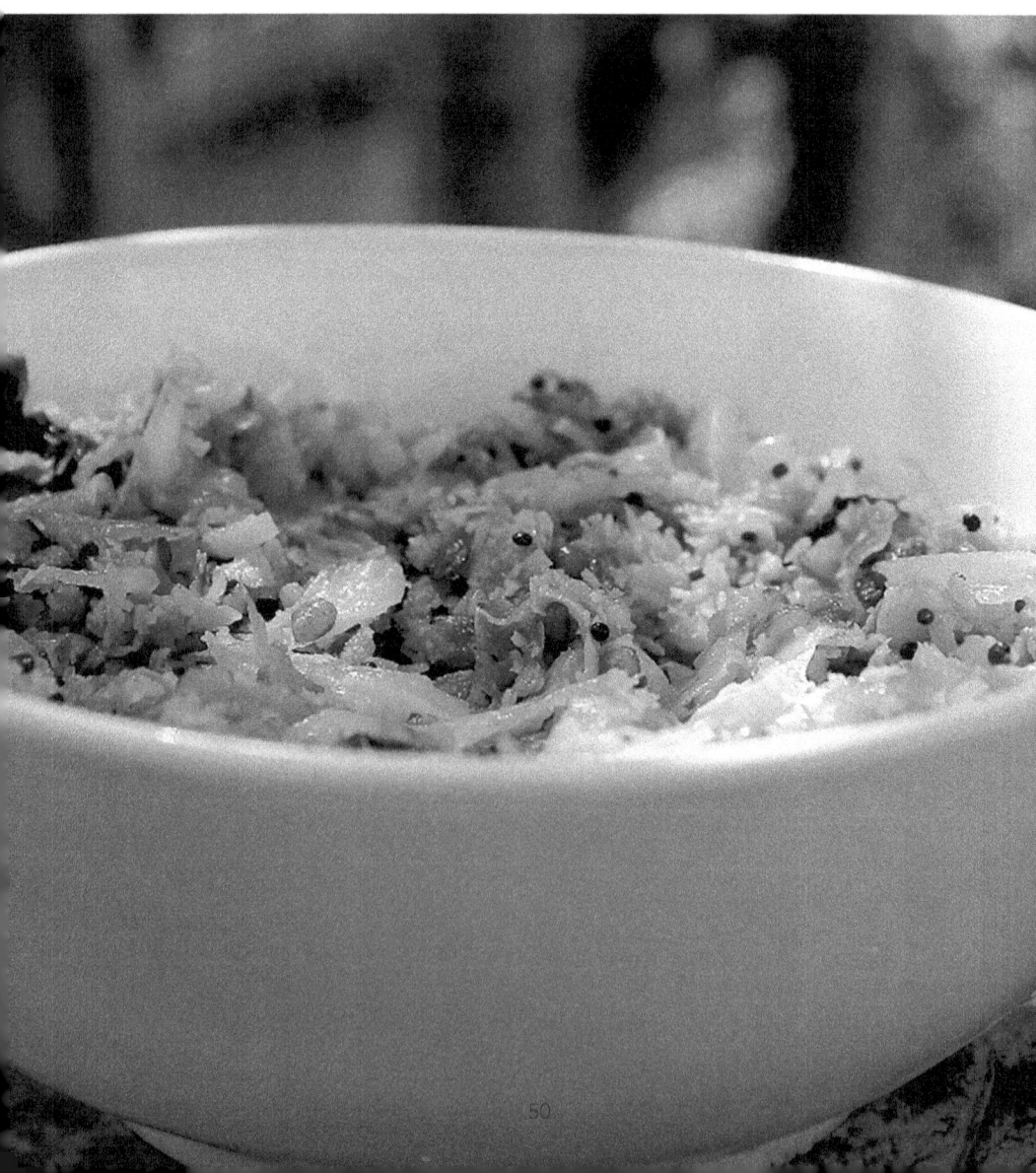

# Carrot Curry

## (MODERATE)

| INGREDIENTS |
| --- |
| • **Carrot (large, sliced);** 1 |
| • **Onion (chopped);** 1/2 |
| • **Green chilli (slit);** 1 |
| • **Curry leaves;** ½ sprig |
| • **Turmeric powder;** 1/4 tsp |
| • **Water;** 1 cup |
| • **Coconut milk powder;** 2 tbsp. |
| • **Lime;** 1/4 |
| • **Salt;** to taste |

## METHOD

1. Cut the carrot into pieces after scraping and washing.

2. Cook the carrot with onion, green chilli, curry leaves, turmeric powder, salt and water.

3. Once the carrot becomes soft, add the coconut milk powder and cook for a few minutes.

4. Remove from stove, add lime and stir.

# Coconut Beans

## (MODERATE)

| INGREDIENTS |
|---|
| • **Beans (Frozen, sliced);** 250 grams |
| • **Coconut flakes (moist);** ½ to 1 cup |
| • **Oil for frying;** 1tbsp. |
| • **Onion;** 1 |
| • **Garlic (minced);** 2 tsp |
| • **Ginger (minced);** 2 tsp |
| • **Curry leaves (sliced);** 1tbsp. |
| • **Mustard seeds;** 2 tsp |
| • **Cumin seeds;** 2 tsp |
| • **Green chilli;** 1 |
| • **Curry powder;** 1 tbsp. |
| • **Salt;** to taste |

## METHOD

1. Chop the onion and green chilli into thin pieces.

2. Pour the oil into the frying pan and heat.

3. Once the oil is hot, add the onions.

4.  When the onions appear translucent add the mustard seeds, cumin seeds, garlic, ginger and curry leaves.

5.  After a couple of minutes, add the beans (250g) and continue frying.

6.  When the beans start to brown, add the curry powder and thoroughly mix.

7.  Continue frying the beans till water is removed and beans are slightly charred.

8.  Add the coconut flakes (half a cup first) and if more is required, depending on taste add the rest of the cup.

9.  Turn off the cook top, mix the coconut flakes well and then add salt as required and serve.

# Dhal with Spinach

## (CHALLENGING)

| INGREDIENTS |
| --- |
| • **Mysore dhal;** 1/2 cup |
| • **Water;** 1/2 cup |
| • **Turmeric;** 1/4 tsp |
| • **Onion (medium, finely chopped);** 1/2 |
| • **Garlic (chopped);** 3 cloves |
| • **Spinach;** 150 grams |
| • **Coconut milk;** 1/4 cup |
| • **Salt and black pepper;** to taste |

## INGREDIENTS FOR TEMPERING

- **Onion;** 1/2 cup
- **Green chillies (slit);** 2
- **Curry leaves;** 1 sprig
- **Mustard seed;** 1 tsp
- **Cumin seeds;** 1 tsp
- **Butter;** 1 tbsp.

## METHOD

1. Wash the dhal, place in a pan, add water and turmeric and bring to boil.

2. Lower the heat and add onion and garlic.

3. When the dhal is cooked add the spinach, cover the pan and let the spinach cook for about 5 minutes on a low heat.

4. Once the spinach has cooked, add the salt and coconut milk and cook on a low heat for another 5-10 minutes.

5. Transfer the dhal mixture to a bowl.

6. In another pan, heat butter and add the onions, chillies, curry leaves, mustard seeds and cumin seeds and temper until onions are golden brown. Add this to the dhal mixture and combine well.

7. Add salt and black pepper powder to taste.

# Drumstick White Curry

## (CHALLENGING)

### INGREDIENTS

- **Drumstick (Murunga) (6 cm pieces, skinned);** 250 grams
- **Prawns (small);** 4
- **Green chillies (slit);** 2
- **Curry leaves;** 1 sprig
- **Turmeric;** 1/4 tsp
- **Coconut (fresh, scraped);** 2 tbsp. (Alternatively, soak desiccated coconut in 1 tbsp. milk)
- **Cumin (powder);** 1 tsp
- **Onion (small, chopped);** 1
- **Water;** 1- 1 ½ cups
- **Lime juice;** 1/2 tsp
- **Salt;** to taste

# METHOD

1. Blend coconut, cumin and onion with little water into a paste.

2. Clean the drum-sticks and cut into 6 cm long pieces and slit them.

3. Cook the drum-sticks, onion, green chillies, curry leaves, salt and turmeric with 1 cup water. (add a few small prawns if desired)

4. Once the drum-sticks are cooked well add the above paste and boil. Remove from heat and add lime juice.

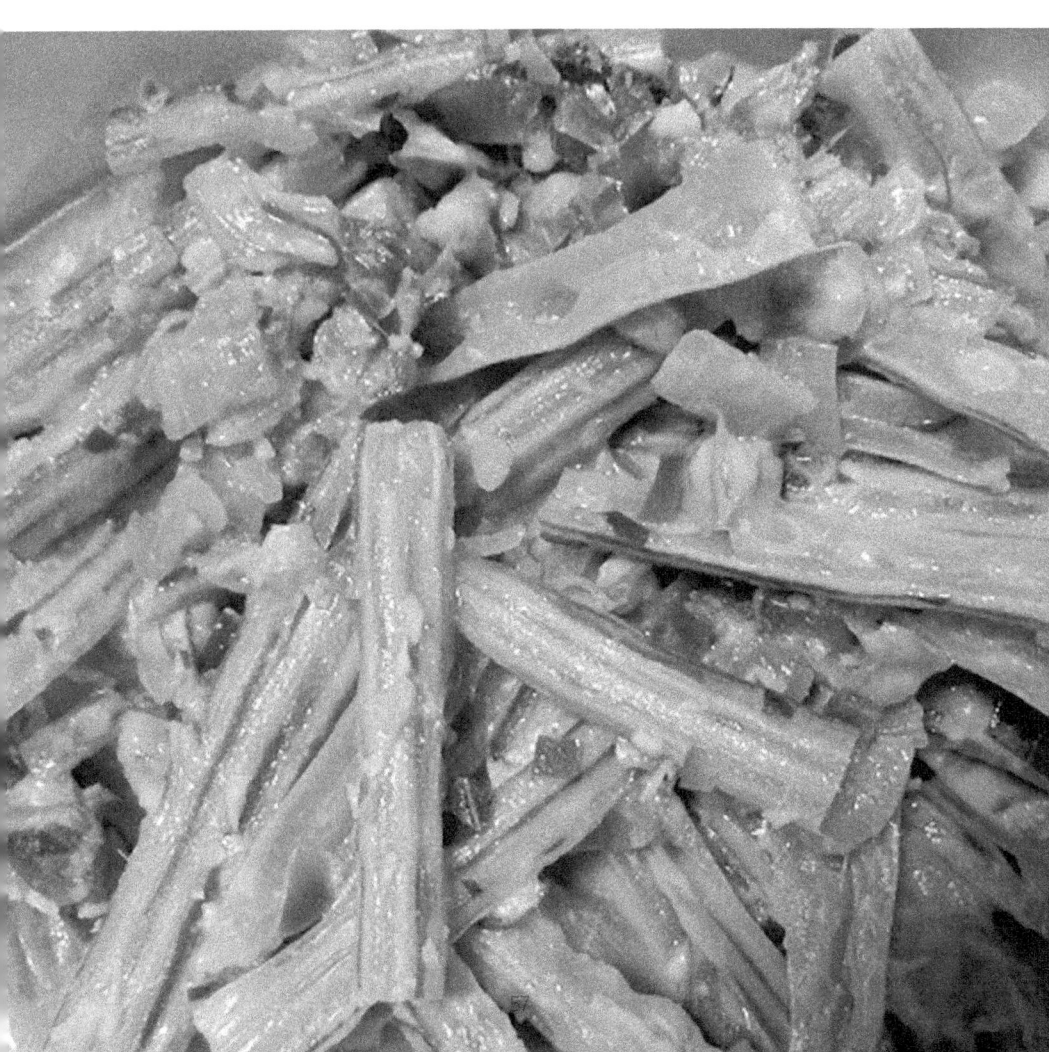

# Drumstick Red Curry

## (CHALLENGING)

| INGREDIENTS |
| --- |

- **Drumstick (Murunga) (cut into pieces);** 250 grams
- **Onion (small, chopped);** 1
- **Garlic (chopped);** 3 cloves
- **Tomato;** 1
- **Green chillies (split);** 2
- **Turmeric;** 1/4 tsp
- **Curry powder;** 2 tsp
- **Fenugreek seeds;** 1/4 tsp
- **Curry leaves;** 1 sprig
- **Milk;** 1/8th cup
- **Sugar (optional);** a pinch
- **Salt;** to taste

## INGREDIENTS FOR TEMPERING

- **Oil;** 2 tbsp.
- **Red chilli (dried, broken into pieces);** 1
- **Onion (very small);** 1
- **Mustard seeds;** 1/4 tsp
- **Curry leaves;** few

# METHOD

1. Clean drumstick and cut into small pieces. Place the drumsticks and all other ingredients except milk in a pan. Add water to cover the drumsticks.

2. Heat until gravy thickens and drumstick is cooked. Add milk and simmer for 5 minutes.

3. In a frying pan put all the ingredients for tempering and heat.

4. When the onion turns golden in colour transfer the contents of the frying pan into the drumstick curry and stir.

5. Add a pinch of sugar to enhance the taste if desired.

# Lentil Curry

## (CHALLENGING)

| INGREDIENTS |
| --- |

- **Red lentils;** ½ cup
- **Water;** 1 cup
- **Dried chillies (broken into pieces);** 1.
- **Turmeric;** 1/4 tsp
- **Oil or ghee;** 1 tbsp.
- **Curry leaves;** 1 sprig
- **Cumin seed;** ½ tsp
- **Mustard seed;** ½ tsp
- **Onion (finely sliced);** 1
- **Garlic (finely sliced);** 2 cloves
- **Milk;** ¼ cup
- **Salt;** to taste

## METHOD

1. Wash the lentils thoroughly and drain.

2. Fill a sauce pan with the drained lentils add enough water to cover the lentils and boil. Discard the froth that forms while boiling. Cook till the lentils are soft.

3. Heat the oil in a frying pan and fry the curry leaves, onions, garlic, chilli, cumin seed and mustard seed and Turmeric until the onions are soft and brown.

4. Transfer this to the lentil mixture. Allow to simmer without covering, for 2 minutes.

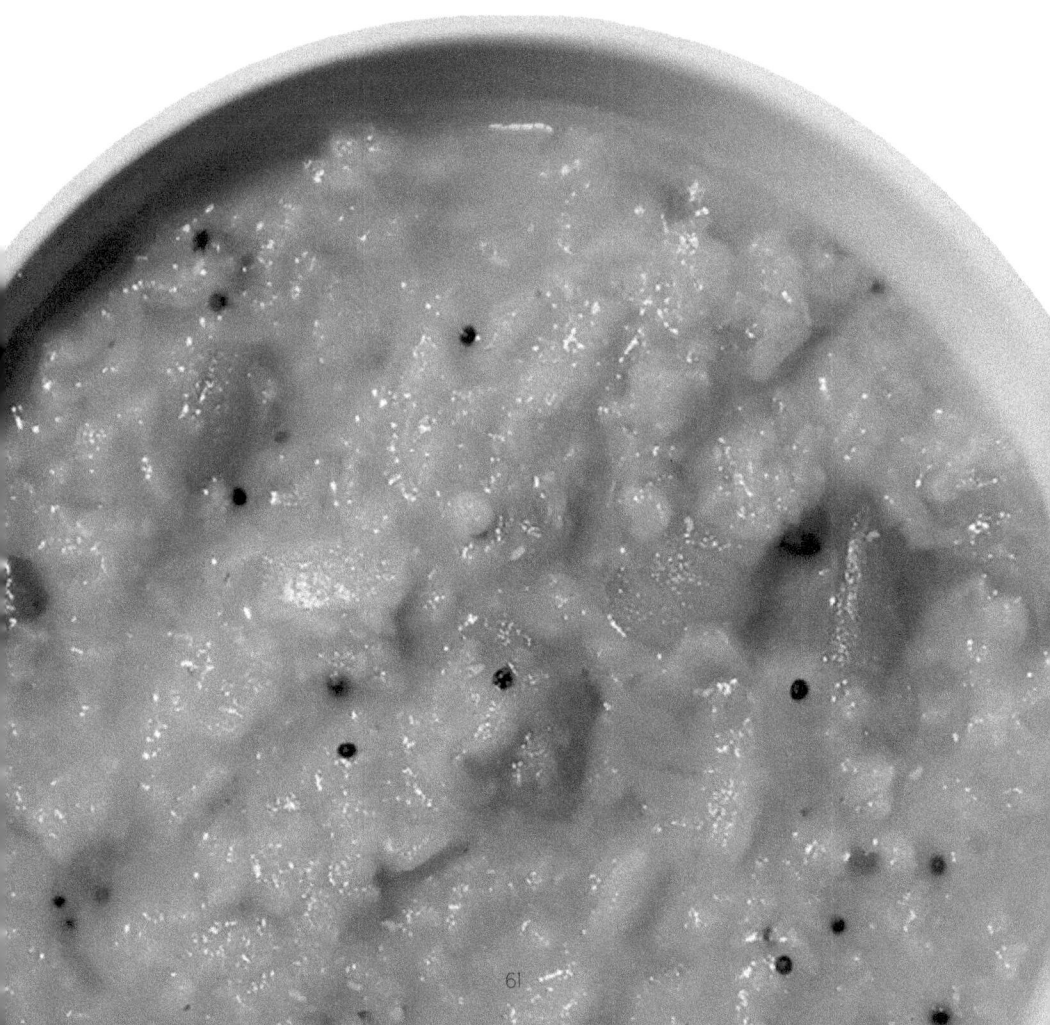

# Long Beans Curry

## (MODERATE)

| INGREDIENTS |
| --- |

- **Long Beans;** 50 grams
- **Oil;** 1 tbsp.
- **Mustard seeds;** a pinch
- **Red onion (sliced);** 1/2
- **Red onion (small, sliced);** 1
- **Chilli powder;** 1/2 tsp
- **Turmeric;** 1/4 - 1/2 tsp
- **Curry powder;** 1 ½ tsp
- **Maldives fish (optional);** 1 tbsp.
- **Coconut (first milk);** 2 tbsp.
- **Coconut (second milk);** 4 tbsp.
- **Salt;** to taste

# METHOD

1. Heat the oil and add mustard seeds (mustard should pop).

2. Add all ingredients except the coconut milk.

3. Cook on medium to high heat for five minutes.

4. Add the second milk and continue to cook, reducing the liquid.

5. Add the first milk just before turning off the heat.

6. Add salt to taste.

**Note:**　**First milk** refers to the milk obtained by squeezing fresh coconut scrapings with water.

**Second milk** is milk obtained by using the squeezed coconut the second time by adding more water.

Canned or powdered coconut could be used instead of fresh coconut milk.

# Mumbai Potato Masala

## (MODERATE)

### INGREDIENTS

- **Potatoes;** 200 grams
- **Butter;** 20 grams
- **Onion (small, sliced);** 1
- **Garlic (crushed);** 2 cloves
- **Mustard seeds;** 1 tsp
- **Curry powder;** 1/2 tbsp.
- **Tomatoes (canned, undrained);** 100 grams

## METHOD

1.  Cut the potatoes into wedges and boil. Set aside

2.  Heat the butter in a large pan and cook in it the onion and garlic stirring until the onion is soft.

3.  Add mustard seeds and curry powder and stir until you get a fragrant smell.

4.  Now add the tomatoes and stir for about 2 minutes or until the sauce thickens slightly.

5.  Add the potatoes and stir gently.

6.  Serve hot.

# Mushroom Curry

## (MODERATE)

### INGREDIENTS

- **Mushroom (cut pieces);** 1 cup
- **Onion;** 1
- **Chilli powder;** 2 tsp
- **Pepper powder;** 2 tsp
- **Garlic (crushed);** 2 cloves
- **Garlic (minced);** 1/2 tbsp.
- **Turmeric;** 1/4 tsp
- **Curry leaves;** 1 sprig
- **Oil;** 1 tbsp.
- **Water;** 2tbsp
- **Salt;** to taste

### METHOD

1. To the mushroom add the pepper powder, chilli powder, turmeric and salt.

2. Mix well and keep aside.

3. Put oil in a saucepan and add the onion and garlic and fry till the onion browns.

4. Add curry leaves and 2 tbsp. water and boil for 1 minute.

5. Add the mushroom and mix well.

6. After a few minutes allow to cool and serve.

# Ladies' Fingers Curry

## (MODERATE)

| INGREDIENTS |
| --- |

- **Ladies' Fingers (Okra) (cut at angle);** 200 grams
- **Mustard seeds;** a pinch
- **Rumpe;** 2 – 3
- **Curry leaves;** 1 sprig
- **Red onion (small, sliced);** 1
- **Chilli flakes;** 1 tbsp.
- **Turmeric;** 1/4 tsp
- **Maldives fish;** 1tbs
- **Oil;** 1 tbsp.
- **Lime;** 1/4
- **Salt;** to taste

# METHOD

1. Heat oil and add mustard seeds (mustard seeds should pop).

2. Add rumpe and curry leaves.

3. Add onion.

4. Add ladies' fingers and stir continuously.

5. Add salt to taste- Add rest of the ingredients.

6. Continue frying until slime dries up.

7. Turn the heat off and add lime juice.

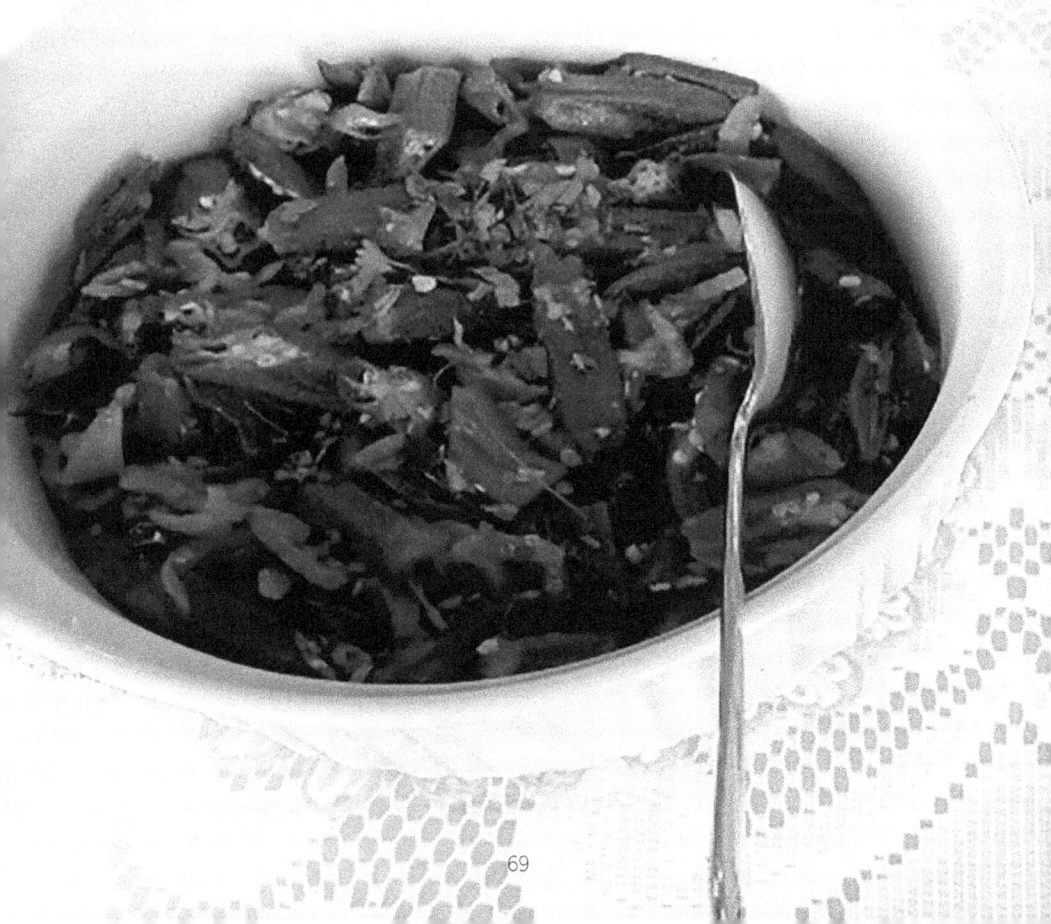

# Pumpkin Curry

## (MODERATE)

| INGREDIENTS |
| --- |

- **Pumpkin (with or without skin);** 200 grams
- **Garlic (pounded);** 1 clove
- **Oil;** 1 tbsp.
- **Mustard seeds;** a pinch
- **White pepper;** a pinch
- **Red onion (sliced);** 1/4
- **Rumpe;** 2 or 3
- **Curry leaves;** 1/2 a sprig
- **Chilli powder;** 1 tsp
- **Coconut milk (first milk);** 1 tbsp.
- **Coconut (second milk);** 2 tbsp.
- **Turmeric;** 1/4 tsp
- **Curry powder;** 1/2 tsp
- **Water;** as required
- **Salt;** to taste

# METHOD

1.  Heat the oil in a pan and add mustard seed.

2.  Add garlic, pepper, onion, rumpe and curry leaves and saute for a few minutes.

3.  Add the pumpkin, salt and water. Cook on medium heat until the pumpkin is tender.

4.  Add chilli powder, turmeric, curry powder and second milk and continue cooking for few minutes.  Add the first milk and stir before taking off the stove.

**Note:**  **First milk** refers to the milk obtained by squeezing fresh coconut scrapings with water.

**Second milk** is milk obtained by using the squeezed coconut the second time by adding more water.

Canned or powdered coconut could be used instead of fresh coconut milk.

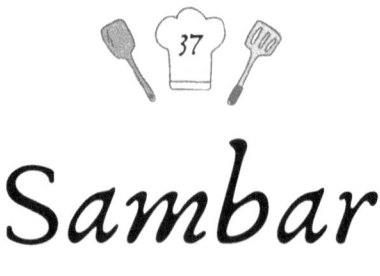

# Sambar

## (MODERATE)

Sambar is a lentil based vegetable stew made with a number of vegetables. It is a good accompaniment for Thosai, Idly, Pittu and String hoppers.

<table>
<tr><th>INGREDIENTS</th></tr>
</table>

- **Sambar powder;** 2 tbsp.
- **Red lentils;** 1/2 cup
- **Red chilli;** 2
- **Onion (large);** 1
- **Potato;** 1
- **Ash plantain;** 1/2 – 1 (optional)
- **Eggplant;** 1/4
- **Carrot; (cut into pieces);** 1
- **Tomato;** 1
- **Curry leaves;** 2 sprigs
- **Garlic;** 1 pod
- **Tamarind paste:** 2 tbsp.
- **Water;** (as required)
- **Salt;** to taste.

# METHOD

1. Boil the red lentil in water. Keep aside.

2. Put all vegetables, curry leaves, tamarind and salt in a pan and cover with water and boil.

3. Once cooked add the lentil and sambar powder and a little milk if desired and simmer for a few minutes.

4. Add tempered onion, mustard seeds, cumin seeds, red chilli & curry leaves to give the sambar some flavour.

# Spinach Curry

## (MODERATE)

| INGREDIENTS |
| --- |

- **Frozen spinach;** 500 grams
- **Onion (medium, chopped);** 1
- **Garlic (finely chopped);** 3 cloves
- **Curry leaves;** 1 sprig
- **Mustard seeds;** 1 tsp
- **Cumin seeds;** 1/2 tsp
- **Turmeric;** 1/4 tsp
- **Milk;** 1/2 cup
- **Green chillies;** 2

## METHOD

1.  Heat oil in a saucepan and add onions, green chillies & garlic
2.  Add mustard seeds, cumin seeds & curry leaves.
3.  Fry until the onions are golden brown and then add turmeric
4.  Add Spinach & salt.

5.  Stir and fry for 2-3 minutes.

6.  Reduce the heat and allow the spinach to cook.

7.  Add coconut milk (or cow's milk) and allow to simmer for a few minutes.

# Zucchini Curry

## (MODERATE)

### INGREDIENTS

- **Zucchini;** 2
- **Oil;** 1 tbsp.
- **Mustard seeds;** 1/4 tsp
- **Cumin seeds;** 1/2 tsp
- **Onion (finely chopped);** 1
- **Chillies (finely chopped);** 2
- **Ginger (small piece, finely chopped);** 1
- **Garlic (sliced);** 2 -3 cloves
- **Garlic (chopped);** 2 cloves
- **Curry powder;** 1 tbsp.
- **Turmeric powder;** 1/4 tsp
- **Fenugreek seeds;** 1/2 tsp
- **Water;** 1/2 cup
- **Coconut milk;** 1/4 cup
- **Sour cream;** 1 tbsp. or as desired
- **Salt;** to taste

# METHOD

1. Wash and slice zucchini.

2. Heat the oil, add the mustard and cumin seeds and cook until mustard starts to pop.

3. Add the onions, green/red chillies, curry leaves, ginger and garlic, and cook for a few minutes until onion turns golden brown.

4. Add curry powder, turmeric powder, and fenugreek seeds.

5. Add the zucchini slices and the water. Bring the gravy to boil and then simmer until zucchini becomes tender.

6. Add the coconut milk and heat till the gravy thickens.

7. Add the sour cream and salt to the gravy at the end.

# *Jasmine's*
# TAMIL
# KITCHEN

## POULTRY AND EGG DISHES

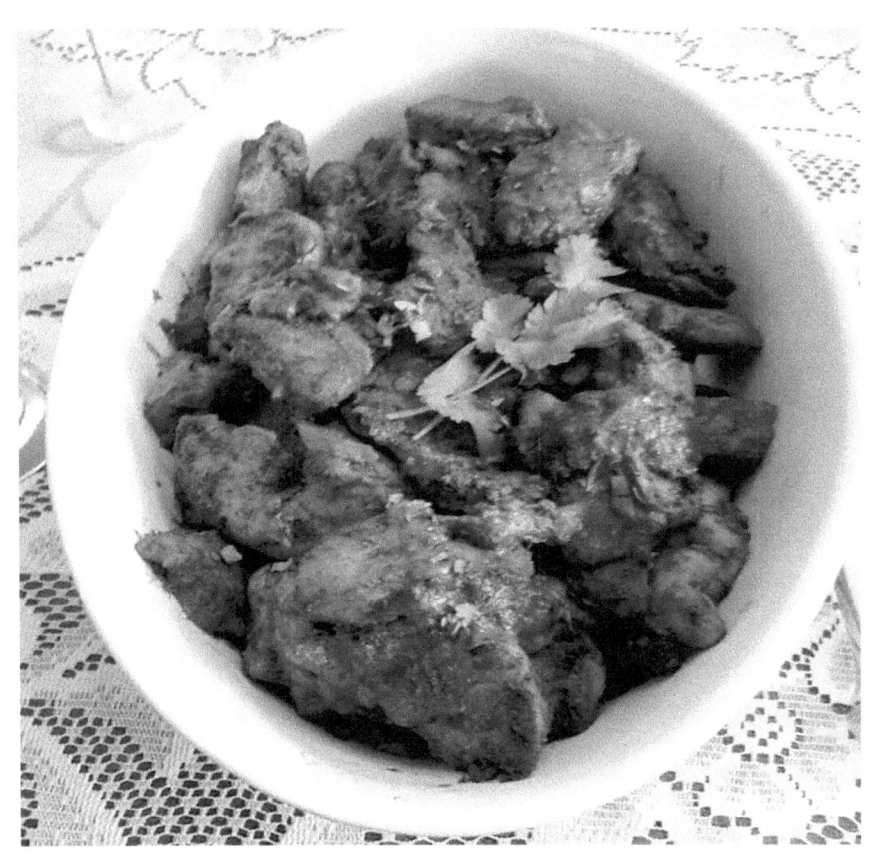

# Apricot Chicken

## (MODERATE)

### INGREDIENTS

- **Chicken breast (small pieces);** 200 grams
- **Olive oil;** 1 tbsp. (2 lots)
- **Butter; –** 1 tbsp. (2 lots)
- **Onions (diced);** 2
- **Bacon (rashers, sliced);** 2
- **Capsicum (red, sliced);** 1
- **Apricot (dried);** 1 cup
- **Paprika;** 1 tsp
- **Flour (white);** 1 tbsp.
- **Sugar (Brown);** 1 tsp
- **Chicken Stock;** 1/2 cup

# METHOD

1.  Fry the chicken pieces in 1 tbsp. olive oil and 1 tbsp. butter till they brown.

2.  Sprinkle the flour and cook for a couple of more minutes. Set aside.

3.  In another pan, cook the onions in oil and butter (1 tbsp. each).

4.  Add the bacon rashers, red capsicum and cook for a couple of more minutes.

5.  Now add the chicken, paprika, apricot, sugar and the chicken stock.

6.  Mix well and bring to boil.

7.  Allow to simmer for 10 minutes.

# Boiled Egg Gravy

## (MODERATE)

| INGREDIENTS |
|---|

- **Eggs (hard boiled);** 3
- **Onion (medium, chopped);** 1
- **Tomato (medium, cut into 4 pieces);** 1
- **Curry leaves (chopped);** 1 sprig
- **Fenugreek seeds;** 1/2 tsp
- **Green chilli (split);** 1
- **Turmeric;** 1/4 tsp
- **Water;** 2 cups
- **Coconut milk (or cow's milk);** 1/2 cup
- **Lime;** 1/4
- **Salt;** to taste

# METHOD

1. Remove the shells from the boiled eggs, lightly slit them and keep aside.

2. Put all the ingredients except the milk and lime in a pan and let it boil for few minutes.

3. Add the eggs and milk and simmer. Add the lime juice

4. Temper the following additional ingredients in 1 tbsp. oil and pour into the gravy: (optional)

    **Finely chopped onion;** ¼

    **Red dry chilli (cut to pieces);** 1

    **Curry leaves;** few

    **Mustard seeds;** ¼ tsp

    **Cumin seeds;** ¼ tsp

# Chicken Curry

## (MODERATE)

| INGREDIENTS |
| --- |

- **Chicken pieces (skinned);** 250 grams
- **Oil;** 1 tsp
- **Onion (chopped);** 1
- **Garlic (chopped);** 2 cloves.
- **Ginger (chopped);** 1 small piece
- **Turmeric;** 1 tsp
- **Curry powder;** 2 tsp
- **Tomato (chopped);** 1
- **Curry leaves;** 1 sprig
- **Water (optional);** 1/2 cup
- **Salt;** to taste

# METHOD

1.  Marinate the chicken with garlic, ginger, turmeric, curry powder, and salt in a large bowl. Mix well and leave for 1 -2 hours.

2.  Heat the oil in a pan, add the onion and fry until golden.

3.  Add tomatoes to the marinated chicken.

4.  Cover and cook for 30 minutes in a low fire until the chicken is tender.

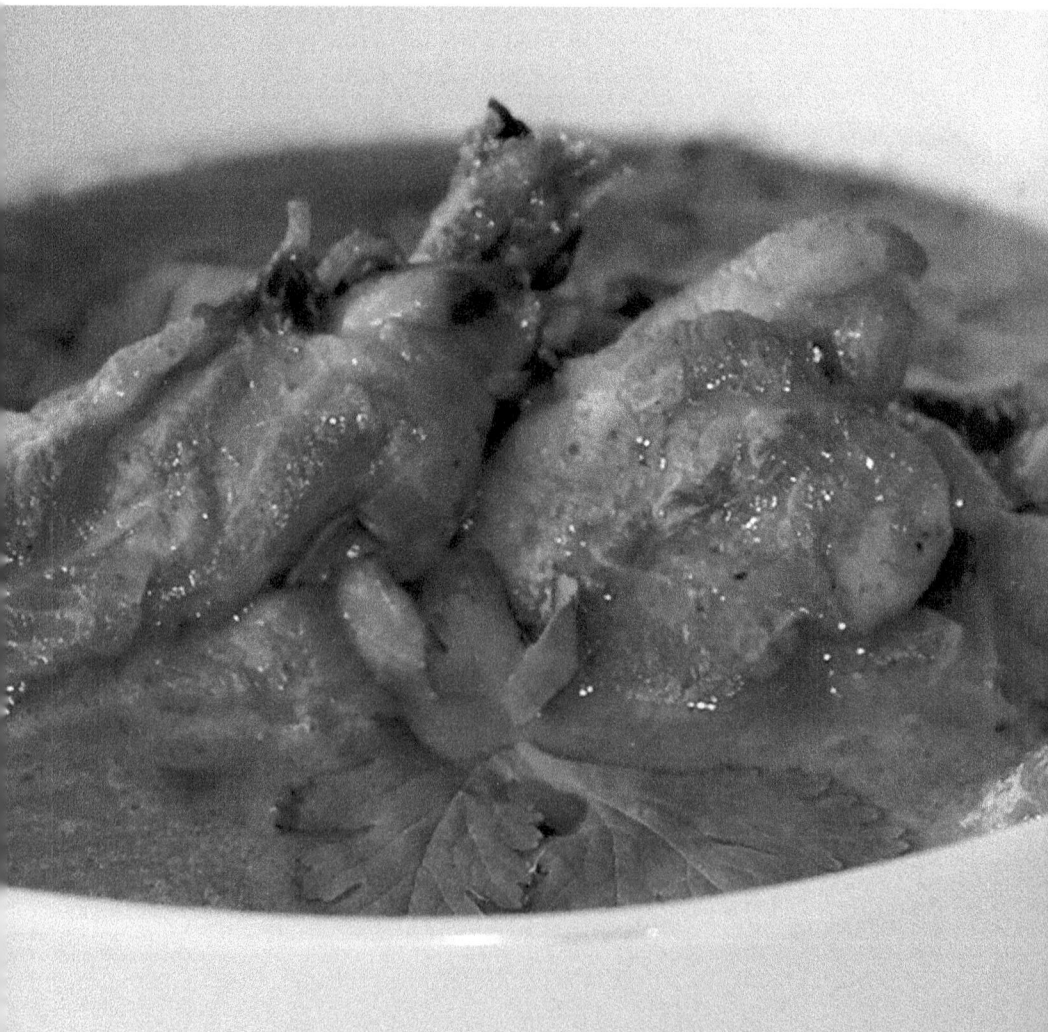

# Chicken Stir Fry

## (CHALLENGING)

| INGREDIENTS |
|---|
| • **Chicken thighs;** 250 grams |
| • **Vegetable Oil;** 3 tbsp. |
| • **Chicken cube;** 1 |
| • **Curry paste;** 2 tbsp. * |
| • **Garlic;** 6 -8 pods |
| • **Garam Masala;** (1/2 -1 tsp) |
| • **Leek;** 1 ** |
| • **Onion (large);** 1 |
| • **Coconut milk (optional);** 1/2 cup |

*Different varieties are available in super markets.

** Cabbage or spinach can be substituted

# METHOD

1. Chop up chicken into small pieces and add one tablespoon of curry paste and leave aside.

2. Chop up the garlic and onion.

3. Heat the oil in a frying pan and when hot add garlic first and then onion and fry. Add the curry paste , chicken, chicken cube and continue to fry with the lid on until chicken is cooked and water from the chicken is absorbed.

4. Add the curry paste , chicken, chicken cube and continue to fry with the lid on until chicken is cooked and water from the chicken is absorbed.

5. When sizzling, add chopped up leek, (or cabbage or spinach] and mix with the chicken till they shrink. Sprinkle garam masala powder and add salt to taste. If preferred, add some coconut milk at this point and mix well.

# Fried Chicken

## (MODERATE)

### INGREDIENTS -1

- **Chicken thighs;** 6 pieces
- **Curry powder;** 1 tsp
- **Ginger (crushed);** 2 small pieces
- **Garlic (crushed);** 3 cloves.
- **Turmeric;** 1/2 tsp
- **Pepper powder;** 1/2 tsp

### INGREDIENTS -2

- **Bread crumbs;** 1/2 cup
- **Curry powder;** 1/2 tsp
- **Black pepper;** 1/2 tsp
- **Corn flour;** 1/4 cup
- **Spice powder;** 1/2 tsp
- **Salt;** 1/2 tsp

# METHOD

1.  Wash the chicken thoroughly after peeling off the skin.

2.  Pierce the chicken with a fork.

3.  Make a paste out of ingredients -1 and coat the chicken with it.

4.  Set it aside for about 6 hours.

5.  Cook the chicken until dry.

6.  Mix ingredients – 2 in a bowl and coat the chicken with it while chicken is very warm.  Fry the chicken until it turns to a dark golden colour.

# Hot and Spicy Chicken Wings

## (EASY)

| INGREDIENTS |
|---|
| • **Chicken wings;** 250 grams |
| • **Ginger (grated);** 1 tsp |
| • **Chilli powder;** 2 tsp |
| • **Oil;** 2 tsp |
| • **Garlic (crushed);** 1 clove |
| • **Vinegar (or sherry);** 2 tbsp. |
| • **Honey;** 1 tbsp. |
| • **Soy sauce;** 1 tbsp. |
| • **Salt and pepper;** as required |

## METHOD

1. Mix all ingredients with chicken and refrigerate overnight.

2. Bake for 35-40 minutes at 200 degrees Celsius

# Omelette

## (EASY)

| INGREDIENTS |
|---|
| • **Eggs**: 2 |
| • **Oil;** 2 tbsp. |
| • **Onion (medium, chopped);** 1 |
| • **Green chillies (chopped);** 2. |
| • **Curry leaves (chopped);** 1 sprig |
| • **Salt and pepper;** to taste |
| • **Spice powder:** ¼ tsp |

## METHOD

1.    Whisk the eggs with spice powder, salt and pepper.

2.    Heat the oil in a non-stick pan.

3.    Fry the onions, green chillies and curry leaves for a few minutes.

4.    Pour the egg mixture slowly to cover the entire inside of the pan.

5.    Cook on medium heat with the lid on.

6.    After few minutes, lift the edge of the omelette to see if it has turned golden; if so turn the other side and cook only for another half a minute.

# Omelette Curry

## (EASY)

| INGREDIENTS |
|---|

- **Omelette (refer to Omelette recipe above);** 1 or 2
- **Oil;** 2 tbsp.
- **Potato (cut into cubes);** 1
- **Onion (medium, chopped);** 1
- **Dry red chilli (broken to pieces);** 1
- **Curry leaves (chopped);** 1 sprig
- **Curry powder;** 1 tbsp.
- **Tamarind paste (thick);** 1/2 tsp
- **Water;** 1 cup
- **Coconut milk ( or cow's milk);** 1/2 cup
- **Salt;** to taste

# METHOD

1. Heat the oil in a pan and fry the potato cubes until they turn to a golden colour.

2. Add the onion, curry leaves, dry red chili and salt and continue to fry till the onions are translucent.

3. Add curry powder, tamarind paste and water and boil.

4. Add the omelette (cut into pieces) and the milk and simmer for a few minutes.

# Ricotta Cheese Curry

## (MODERATE)

| INGREDIENTS |
|---|
| • **Ricotta cheese;** 500 grams |
| • **Eggplant;** 100 to 150 grams |
| • **Oil for frying** |
| • **Tomatoes;** 2 |
| • **Onion;** 1 |
| • **Curry leaves;** 9 |
| • **Chilli powder;** 2 tbsp. |
| • **Water;** 2 cups |
| • **Fenugreek seeds;** ½ tsp |
| • **Garlic Cloves (sliced);** 6 |
| • **Salt;** to taste |

# METHOD

1. Chop the onion into small pieces.

2. Cut the cheese into 2 cm cubes.

3. Cut the eggplant into 1.5 cm cubes.

4. Add oil to the frying pan and heat.

5. Fry cheese pieces and eggplant separately until golden brown and then keep aside.

6. Fry the onion till it browns and add garlic, fenugreek seeds and curry leaves.

7. After 2 minutes, add chilli powder, tomato, fried cheese, fried eggplant and water.

8. Boil for 10 minutes, stirring occasionally until a thicker curry consistency develops.

9. Add salt as required and serve.

# Jasmine's
# TAMIL
# KITCHEN

## BEEF, LAMB AND PORK DISHES

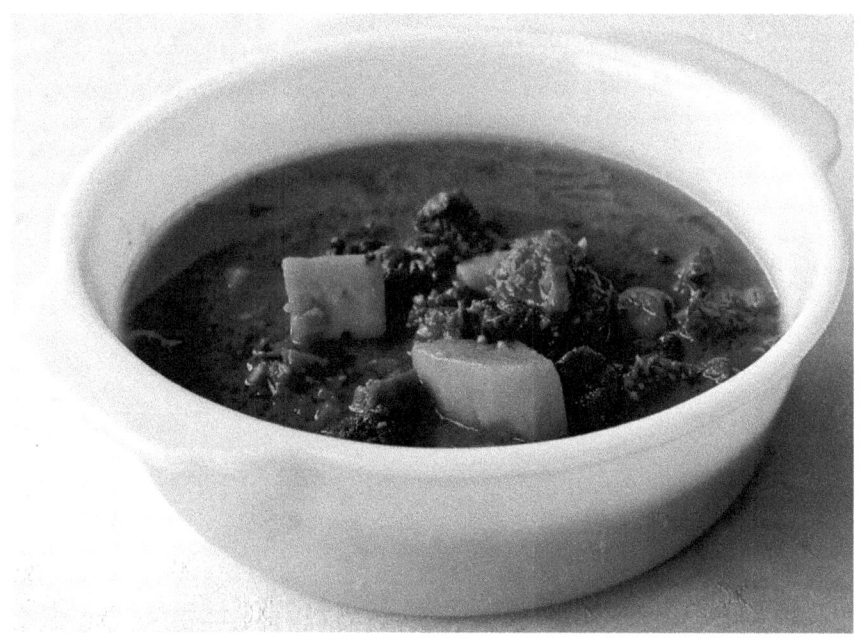

# Beef Curry

## (MODERATE)

| INGREDIENTS |
|---|
| • **Beef (cut into small pieces);** 200 grams |
| • **Oil (or ghee);** 2 tbsp. |
| • **Onion (medium);** 1 |
| • **Ginger (finely chopped);** 1 tsp |
| • **Garlic (finely chopped);** 1 or 2 cloves |
| • **Mustard seeds;** 1/2 tsp |
| • **Fennel seeds;** 1/2 tsp |
| • **Curry leaves;** 1 sprig |
| • **Curry powder;** 1 tbsp. |
| • **Turmeric;** 1 tsp |
| • **Salt;** to taste |

# METHOD

1. Heat oil and gently fry onions, ginger and garlic. When half fried add mustard, fennel and curry leaves until just beginning to turn golden.

2. Add the meat and stir well. Then add curry powder, turmeric, salt and little water if curry is too thick, and stir well.

3. Cover the pan and simmer on low heat until the meat is tender. When tender, add one teaspoonful of spice powder and stir.

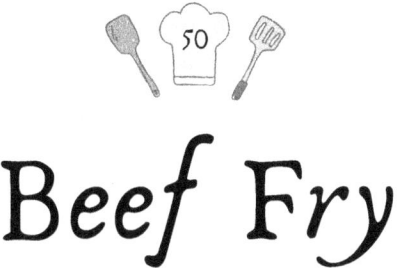

# Beef Fry

## (MODERATE)

| INGREDIENTS |
| --- |

- **Beef (cut into small pieces);** 250 grams
- **Chilli powder (roasted);** 1 tbsp.
- **Ginger paste;** 1 tsp
- **Garlic paste;** 1 tsp
- **Turmeric powder:** 1/2 tsp
- **Onion (thinly sliced);** 1
- **Lemon juice;** 1 tbsp.
- **Oil;** 1 tbsp.
- **Curry leaves;** 1 sprig
- **Salt;** 1 tsp

## METHOD

1. Add salt, turmeric powder, ginger and garlic paste to the cut beef pieces and mix; leave it for 10 minutes.

2. In a pan cook the prepared meat with little water on medium heat.

3.  Add the oil when all the water that came out of the meat dries up.

4.  When it is half fried add the sliced onions and curry leaves and keep frying.

5.  When the onions are fried add chilli powder and mix it for a minute

6.  Add lemon juice and stir.

# Corned Beef Fry

## (EASY)

<table>
<tr><th colspan="2">INGREDIENTS</th></tr>
</table>

- **Corned Beef;** 1 can
- **Onion (small);** 1
- **Curry leaves);** 3 or 4
- **Green chilli;** 1
- **Mustard seeds;** 1/4 tsp
- **Cumin seeds;** 1/4 tsp
- **Lemon juice;** 1 tsp
- **Oil;** 1 tsp
- **Salt and pepper;** to taste

## METHOD

1. Heat the oil in a pan and add the mustard.

2. Add the onion, curry leaves, chilli and cumin.

3. Cook till the onions are soft.

4. Reduce heat and add the corned beef, mix well, and cook for 3 minutes.

5.    Add lemon juice, pepper and salt to taste.

6.    Mix well, put the lid on the pan, and heat for two more minutes.

7.    Enjoy with toast.

# *Lamb Curry*

## (MODERATE)

| INGREDIENTS |
|---|
| • **Lamb;** 200 grams |
| • **Onion (Chopped);** 1 |
| • **Cumin seeds;** 1 tsp |
| • **Oil;** 1 tsp |
| • **Fenugreek seeds;** 1 tsp |
| • **Fennel seeds;** 1/4 tsp |
| • **Curry leaves;** 1 sprig |
| • **Cardamom;** *2* |
| • **Green chilli (small);** 1/2 |
| • **Cinnamon;** 1 stick |
| • **Turmeric;** ½ tsp |
| • **Spice powder;** 1 tsp |
| • **Tomatoes (chopped);** 2 |
| • **Garlic (crushed);** 3 cloves |
| • **Ginger (crushed);** 1 small piece |
| • **Milk;** 1 tbsp. (or as desired) |
| • **Potato (cut into pieces);** 1 |
| • **Curry powder;** 1 ½ tsp |
| • **Tamarind juice;** 1/2 tsp |
| • **Red onion (chopped);** 1 small |
| • **Lemon;** 1 tbsp. |

# METHOD

1. Heat oil in a pot and add onion.

2. Add fennel, cumin, fenugreek, curry leaves, cinnamon, cardamom and green chilli when onion is half cooked.

3. Once the onion turns golden brown add spice powder, turmeric, curry powder, ginger, garlic, tamarind juice and mix well.

4. Add tomatoes and stir the mixture in the pot until it becomes a paste.

5. Add the lamb, stir and cook on high heat for 5 mins.

6. Reduce heat and add in potato. When the potato is cooked sprinkle red onions and leave for 5 minutes.

7. After 10 mins add milk and stir. After a further 5 mins add lemon and stir.

# Meat with Aubergine

## (CHALLENGING)

### INGREDIENTS

- **Minced Lamb or Beef;** 250 grams
- **Aubergine/ Eggplant;** 1
- **Potato (medium size);** 1
- **Onion (medium, chopped);** 1
- **Oil;** 2 tbsp.
- **Garlic (finely chopped);** 2 cloves
- **Tomato (chopped);** 1
- **Tomato puree;** 1 tbsp.
- **Roasted Curry powder;** 1 tsp
- **Ground cinnamon;** 1/2 tsp
- **Cheese (grated);** 100 grams
- **Lemon juice, pepper and salt;** to taste

# METHOD

1. Heat 1 tbsp. oil in a large sauté pan, add the onion and garlic. Stir fry until it turns golden.

2. Add the meat and cook until the liquid is evaporated. Stir in the Cinnamon, chopped tomatoes, tomato puree and cook for 30 mins. Set aside.

3. Peel the Potato and microwave for 3 mins. Or boil to a consistency to be able to slice. Slice Aubergine at an angle or length wise and sprinkle with salt and lemon juice. Set aside.

4. Make a thick white sauce in a pan at low heat continuously stirring and beating the following ingredients without letting to cake.

5. **Flour;** 2 tbsp. **Butter or Margarine;** ½ tbsp. **and milk;** approx. 2 cups (and water if needed)

6. Spread 2 spoons of oil on the bottom of an oven proof dish. Lay the cooked sliced potato then spread half of the meat mixture. Lay the sliced Aubergine slightly overlapping to cover the dish. Spread the rest of the meat mixture. Sprinkle 1/3rd of the grated cheese

7. Pour the prepared white sauce. Sprinkle the rest of the grated cheese. Bake at 180 degree Celsius for 1 hr until bubbling and golden.

8. Allow the dish to cool for 10 mins. Before serving.

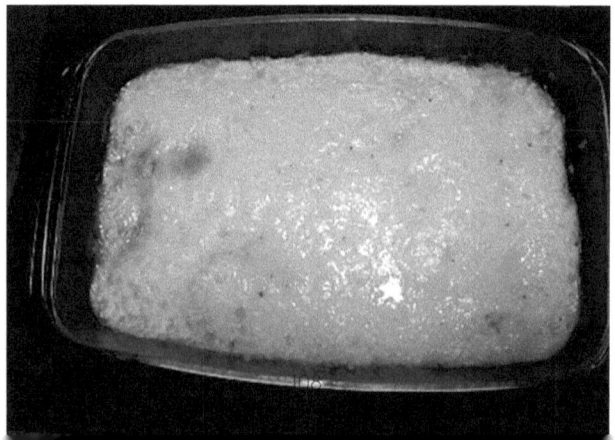

# Meat With Vegetables

## (MODERATE)

| INGREDIENTS |
|---|

- **Lamb or Beef (Minced);** 250 grams
- **Mixed vegetables (frozen);** 250 grams
- **Onion (medium, chopped);** 1
- **Oil;** 1 tbsp.
- **Garlic (finely chopped);** 2 cloves
- **Tomato (chopped);** 1 can
- **Tomato puree;** 2 tbsp.
- **Curry leaves;** 1 sprig
- **Roasted Curry powder;** 1 ½ tsp
- **Cinnamon (ground);** ½ tsp
- **Cumin seed;** ½ tsp
- **Mustard seed;** ½ tsp
- **Salt and Pepper;** to taste

# METHOD

1. Put 1 tbsp. oil in a sauté pan, add the onion and fry until it turns golden.

2. Add the mustard, Cumin, curry leaves and garlic. Add the meat and cook until the liquid is evaporated.

3. Add the chopped tomato and frozen vegetables and cover and cook until the vegetables are cooked.

4. Stir in the curry powder, cinnamon powder and tomato puree and cook for 10 mins.

5. Add salt and pepper.

# Mutton and Peas Curry

## (MODERATE)

| INGREDIENTS |
| --- |

- **Mutton;** 500 grams
- **Green peas;** 500 grams
- **Ghee or butter;** 2 tbsp.
- **Flour (white);** 1 tbsp.
- **Onion (sliced);** 1/2
- **Lime juice;** 1 tbsp.
- **Water;** 3 cups
- **Salt;** to taste

Make a masala paste by grinding;

- **Onion;** 1
- **Pepper corns;** 4
- **Fennel seeds;** 1 tsp
- **Coconut chip;** 1 small piece
- **Coriander leaves;** a few

# METHOD

1. Cut, wash and cook the meat in 3 cups of water.

2. Add the green peas and boil till the peas are cooked.

3. Heat the ghee or butter in another pan, fry the onion in it, sprinkle the flour and stir.

4. When onion is browned add the meat/ pea mixture, the masala paste and salt.

5. Add lemon juice and simmer for 15 minutes.

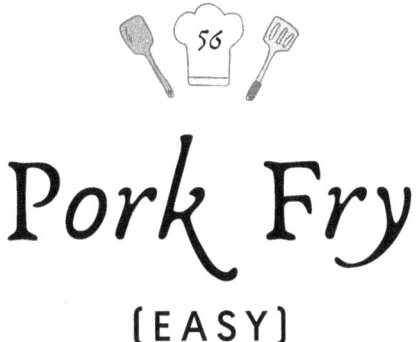

# Pork Fry

## (EASY)

---

### INGREDIENTS

- **Pork (cut into cubes);** 200 grams
- **Turmeric powder;** 1/4 tsp.
- **Vinegar;** 2 tsp
- **Onion (thinly sliced);** 1
- **Curry leaves;** 1 sprig
- **Dry red chilli (cut into pieces);** 2
- **Fennel seeds;** 1/4 tsp
- **Curry powder (roasted);** 2 tsp
- **Lime juice;** 2 tsp
- **Salt;** to taste

---

## METHOD

1. Mix turmeric, vinegar and salt with pork and keep for half an hour.

2. Transfer this to a pan and cook with lid on, on medium heat. Water will appear. Stir and let it cook (with lid on) till the water is all absorbed.

3.  Oil will come from the meat. Keep on frying till golden, stirring in between to stop burning. (If oil does not appear, add little oil)

4.  Add onion and curry leaves and continue frying till onion is translucent.

5.  d dry red chilli and fennel seeds and fry for a few minutes and then add roasted curry powder and mix well.

6.  Fry for a further few minutes and add salt as required. Remove from fire and add lime juice.

# Pork Curry

## (MODERATE)

| INGREDIENTS |
| --- |

- **Pork;** 200 grams
- **Onion;** 1
- **Ginger (crushed);** 1 small piece
- **Pepper powder;** 1 tsp
- **Mint leaves;** a few
- **Vinegar;** 2 tbsp.
- **Sugar;** 2 tsp
- **Carrots;** 100 grams
- **Ghee;** 1 tbsp.
- **Boiling water;** 2 cups
- **Salt;** to taste

## METHOD

1.  Cut the pork into small pieces and wash.

2.  Slice the onion, ginger and carrots.

3.  Heat the ghee in a pan and add a little onion and ginger.

4.    Add the pork, salt, vinegar and pepper powder. Close the lid.

5.    When the pork is browned add two cups of boiling water.

6.    Cook for about 1 hour till the meat is soft.

7.    Add the remaining onion, mint and carrots.

8.    When the carrots are soft add sugar. Cook till the gravy is thick.

# *Jasmine's*
# TAMIL
# KITCHEN

## SEAFOOD DISHES

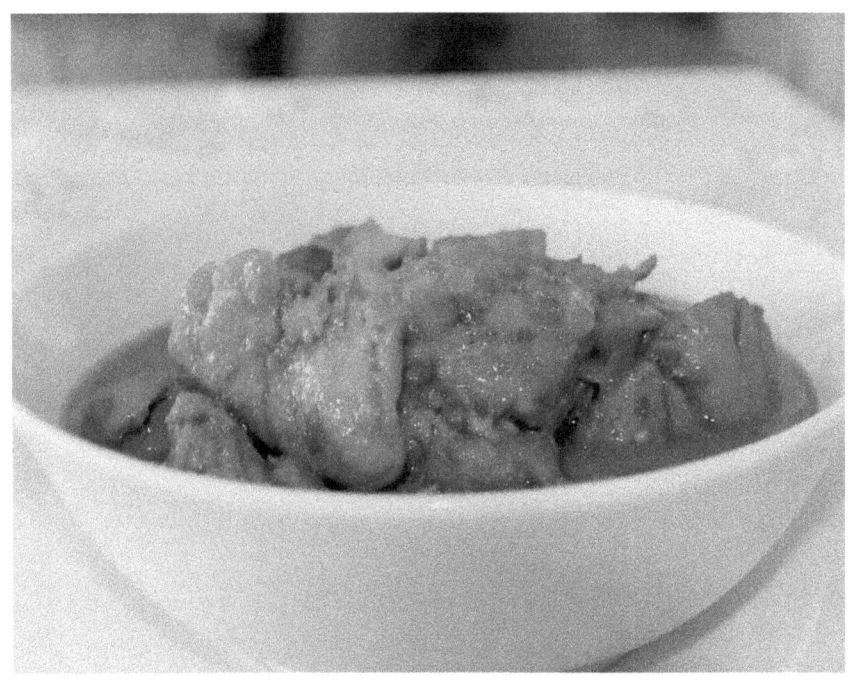

# Crab Curry

## (CHALLENGING)

### INGREDIENTS

- **Crab (cleaned);** 250 grams
- **Turmeric powder;** 1/2 tsp.
- **Curry powder;** 1 ½ tsp
- **Tamarind paste;** 2 tbsp.
- **Oil;** 1 tbs.
- **Onion (big);** 1
- **Garlic (sliced);** 4 pods
- **Curry leaves;** 1 sprig
- **Cumin seeds;** 1 tbs.
- **Green chilli;** 1
- **Coconut milk;** 1/2 cup

### METHOD

1. Mix salt, turmeric powder, curry powder, tamarind paste and coat the crab and keep aside for 10 minutes.

2. In a medium sized pan, fry onions, curry leaves, garlic and cumin seeds in oil. Then add the green chilli and salt.

3.   Once onions turn golden add the crab mixture and cook with lid on for a few minutes.

4.   Finally add the coconut milk and simmer for a few more minutes.

# Cutlets (Fish/ Crab/Prawn)

## (CHALLENGING)

| INGREDIENTS |
| --- |

- **Fish or crab meat or prawns (cooked and mashed);** 200 grams
- **Potato (Boiled and mashed);** 100 grams
- **Oil:** 2 tbsp.
- **Onion (Chopped) medium;** 1
- **Green chillies (chopped);** 2
- **Curry leaves (chopped);** 1 sprig
- **Garlic paste;** 1 tsp
- **Ginger paste;** 1tsp
- **Cumin seeds;** 1 tsp
- **Turmeric powder;** ¼ tsp
- **Curry powder;** 1tbsp.
- **Lime juice;** to taste
- **Salt and pepper;** to taste

For coating and frying:

- **Bread crumbs**
- **Eggs; 2**
- **Oil for frying**

# METHOD

1. Heat the oil in a non-stick pan.

2. Fry the onions, green chillies, curry leaves, garlic and ginger pastes, cumin seeds and turmeric powder till the onions are translucent.

3. Add curry powder, salt and pepper and mix well.

4. Add the fish (or crab or prawns) and potatoes and combine together.

5. Add lime juice.

6. Remove from heat and let it cool down.

7. Make round or oval shaped cutlet balls of desired shape..

8. Whisk the eggs in a bowl and put the bread crumbs in another bowl.

9. Dip the cutlet balls in beaten egg and then coat in bread crumbs. (Repeat the process once more to get a crispy coating when fried).

10. Deep fry the cutlets.

# Cuttle Fish Curry

## (CHALLENGING)

| INGREDIENTS |
| --- |

- **Cuttle fish;** 500 grams
- **Onion (chopped);** 1
- **Roasted curry powder;** 1 tbsp.
- **Tamarind juice;** ½ cup
- **Turmeric powder;** ¼ tsp
- **Cinnamon;** 1 small stick
- **Garlic (chopped);** 3 cloves
- **Ginger (chopped);** 1 tbsp.
- **Curry leaves;** a few
- **Fenugreek;** ½ tsp
- **Cumin;** ½ tsp
- **Coconut milk;** ½ cup
- **Salt;** to taste

# METHOD

1. Wash and cut the cuttle fish. Add turmeric and salt. Mix and set aside.

2. Saute the onion in a frying pan, add Fenugreek, cumin, cinnamon, curry leaves, ginger, and garlic and stir fry until the onion turns golden.

3. Add the cuttle fish, cover and cook in low heat until the cuttle fish is cooked.

4. Stir in the curry powder and tamarind juice.

5. Cook for a few more minutes.

6. Add coconut milk and water if more gravy is preferred.

# Fish Curry

## (MODERATE)

| INGREDIENTS |
|---|
| • **Fish (cut into medium cubes);** 200 grams |
| • **Garlic (crushed);** 2 cloves |
| • **Ginger (crushed);** 1 small piece |
| • **Cinnamon (powder);** 1/4 stick |
| • **Tomato (small);** 1 |
| • **Curry peppers (long);** 2 |
| • **Red onion (small, sliced);** 1 |
| • **Curry leaves;** 1 sprig |
| • **Rumpe;** 2 |
| • **Tamarind juice;** 2 tbsp. |
| • **Curry powder;** 1 tsp |
| • **Turmeric;** 1/4 tsp |
| • **Chilli powder;** 1 tbsp. |
| • **Coconut milk (first milk);** 2 tbsp. |
| • **Coconut milk (second milk);** 4 tbsp. |

# METHOD

1. Pound garlic, ginger, and cinnamon and mix with fish and the rest of ingredients including second milk (enough to give small amount of sauce).

2. Heat (medium to high) for 10-20 mins until sauce thickens. Add the first milk just before removing from heat.

# Fish Stir Fry

## (EASY)

| INGREDIENTS |
| --- |

- **Smoked cod;** 250 grams
- **Onion;** 1
- **Garlic;** 2-3 pods
- **Green curry paste;** 2 tbsp.
- **Coconut milk;** 3 tbsp.
- **Vegetable oil;** 2 tbsp.
- **Mustard seeds;** 1/2 tsp
- **Fenugreek seeds;** 1/2 tsp

## METHOD

1. Fry the fenugreek seeds and mustard seeds in oil in a large frying pan.

2. Add garlic pods and onion and fry further.

3. Add the smoked cod, green curry paste and 2tbsp. coconut milk and cook.

4. When cooked add 1 tbsp. of coconut milk and close with lid and turn off the heat.

# Fried Fish

## (EASY)

| INGREDIENTS |
| --- |
| • **Fish fillets;** 2 |
| • **Oil for frying;** as required |
| • (For deep frying or shallow frying) |
| • **Seasoning ingredients** |
| • **Lemon juice;** 1 tsp |
| • **Turmeric powder**; ½ tsp |
| • **Chilli powder;** ½ tsp |
| • **Salt;** ½ tsp |

## METHOD

1. Mix the seasoning ingredients in a bowl.
2. Coat the fish fillets with the seasoning mix.
3. Cover and leave for 30 minutes.
4. Heat the oil in a pan, lay the fish fillets and cook for 2 minutes.
5. Turn the fillets and cook for another 2 minutes.
6. (Depending on the thickness of the fillets, the frying time could be varied).

# Prawn Curry

## (EASY)

| INGREDIENTS |
| --- |
| • **Prawns (cleaned);** 200 grams |
| • **Red chillies (soaked in hot water);** 6 |
| • **Onion (large);** 1 |
| • **Tamarind juice (thick);** 1 tbsp. |
| • **Oil;** 1 tbsp. |
| • **Sugar;** 1 tsp |
| • **Milk;** (as required) |
| • **Salt;** to taste |

## METHOD

1. Grind the chillies and the onion to make a paste.
2. Heat the oil and add the paste.
3. Allow to cook till the oil floats on top.
4. Add the cleaned prawns and cook for 5 to 10 minutes
5. Add the sugar, salt and tamarind.
6. If the curry is too hot add milk as required.

# Prawn Curry

## (MODERATE)

### INGREDIENTS

- **Prawns (green);** 200 grams
- **Curry powder;** 1 tbsp.
- **Oil or ghee;** 1 tbsp.
- **Curry leaves;** 1 sprig
- **Onion (sliced);** 1
- **Garlic (sliced);** 2 cloves
- **Green chilli (split);** 1
- **Fenugreek seeds;** 1 tsp
- **Tamarind juice;** 1 tbsp.
- **Coconut milk;** 1/2 cup
- **Salt;** to taste

## METHOD

1.   Clean the prawns, wash well and in a bowl marinate it with curry powder and salt and keep aside for 20 minutes.

2.  Heat some oil or ghee in a saucepan and add the curry leaves, onions and garlic. Cook until the onions are translucent and add the marinated prawns, green chili and fenugreek seeds.

3.  Stir fry briefly to coat the prawns, then add tamarind juice and continue to cook for further 3 minutes.

4.  Add coconut milk, simmer for 8–10 minutes till prawns are cooked. (Do not cook for too long as the prawns will become rubbery)

# Shrimp Stir Fry

## (EASY)

| INGREDIENTS |
|---|

- **Shrimp (peeled, uncooked, jumbo);** 500 grams
- **Oil;** 3 tbsp.
- **Cashew nuts;** 1/4 cup
- **Ginger (grated);** 1 tsp
- **Onion (medium, finely chopped);** 1
- **Garlic (minced);** 1/2 tbsp.
- **Spinach (washed, shredded);** 200 grams
- **Soy sauce;** 2 tbsp.
- **Chilli powder;** 2 -3 tbs.
- **Curry leaves;** 1 sprig
- **Salt;** to taste

# METHOD

1. Heat oil in a pan and add the cashew nuts. Cook on low heat, stirring continuously until lightly browned. Remove with a slotted spoon and drain on paper towels.

2. Add the shrimp to the oil remaining in the pan and heat until the shrimp turns pink.

3. Add the ginger, chilli powder, garlic, curry leaves and onion. Cook for a few minutes on moderately high heat.

4. Add the spinach and stir-fry briefly. Add the soy sauce, stir in the cashew nuts and serve immediately.

# Tandoori Fish

## (MODERATE)

| INGREDIENTS |
|---|
| • **Cod fish;** 1 |
| • **Oil;** 2 tbsp. |
| • **Lemon juice;** 2 tbsp. |
| • **Ginger;** 1 small piece |
| • **Garlic flakes;** 7 |
| • **Green chillies;** 5 |
| • **Yoghurt;** 1/2 cup |
| • **Red colouring;** 5 drops |
| • **Salt;** to taste |

***Make a powder of the following;***

Garam masala 1/2 tsp ; coriander seeds (roasted) 1 tsp ; cumin seeds (roasted); 1tsp;  Red chilli powder1/2 tsp ; Dry red chillies 2; Turmeric powder 1 tsp;

# METHOD

1.  Clean the fish. Remove gills and eyes. Cut slits on both sides of the fish.

2.  Apply salt and lemon juice over the fish. Keep aside for 1/2 hour. Grind green chillies, ginger and garlic to a paste. Beat yoghurt thoroughly.

3.  Add ground spices and ginger-garlic paste. Add oil, colour and strain through fine sieve. Rub the batter all over the fish and well inside the slits.

4.  Keep aside for 5-6 hours. Place the fish in tandoor. Remove when golden brown. Ready to serve hot.

**Note:** A Tandoor is a cylindrical clay or metal oven used in cooking and baking.

# *Jasmine's*
# TAMIL
# KITCHEN

## CHUTNEY, PICKLES, AND SAMBOLS

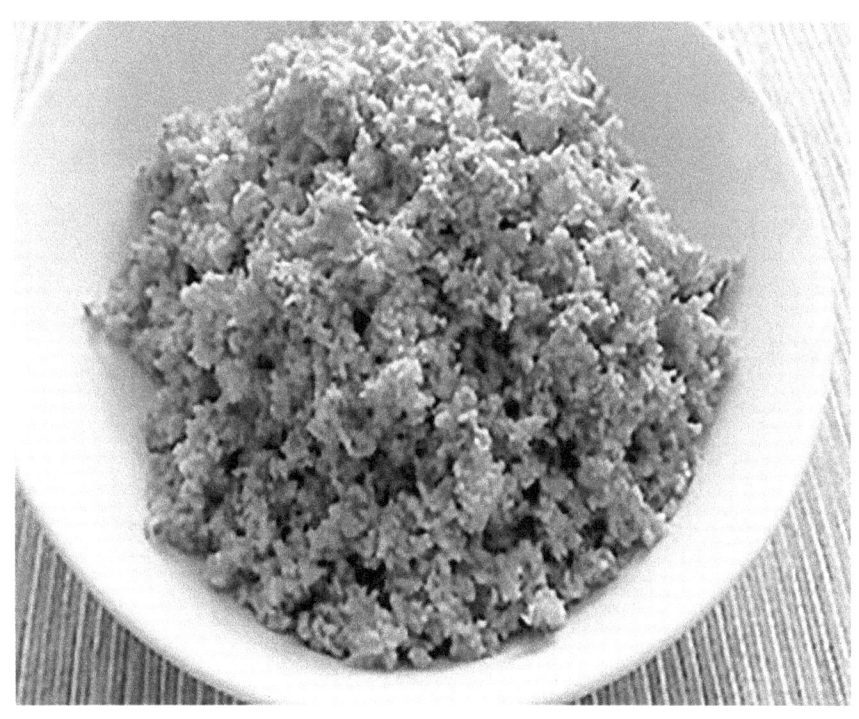

# Aubergine Pickle

## (EASY)

### INGREDIENTS

- **Aubergine (eggplant);** 500 grams
- **Onions (small);** 1 (or 15 shallots)
- **Green chilies;** 10
- **Curry leaves;** 2 sprigs
- **Garlic;** 1 pod
- **Oil;**( for frying)
- **Vinegar;** 4 tbsp.
- **Chilli powder (raw);** 2 tbsp.
- **Sugar;** 2 tbsp.

### METHOD

1. Fry the first five ingredients.

2. In another pan put the last three ingredients and bring to boil.

3. Transfer the fried ingredients to this pan and toss (don't mix with spoon).

# Aubergine Sambol

## (EASY)

| INGREDIENTS |
| --- |

- **Aubergine (eggplant) (medium size);** 1
- **Onion (medium);** 1
- **Ginger (scraped);** 1 small piece
- **Mustard (ground);** 1/4 tsp
- **Chilli powder;** 1 tsp
- **Curry leaves;** 1 sprig
- **Tamarind juice (thick);** 1 tbsp.
- **Coconut milk;** 1 tbsp.
- **Oil (for deep frying and tempering);** as required
- **Salt;** to taste

# METHOD

1. Cut the eggplant into small cubes, wash well and rub with salt and a little turmeric powder.

2. Deep fry the eggplant in oil until golden brown. Keep aside.

3. Slice the onion thinly and deep fry in oil. Keep aside.

4. Warm 1½ tsp oil in another pan and temper ginger, mustard, curry leaves and chilli powder until aromatic.

5. Add tamarind juice, the fried eggplant and fried onion, and mix well, and simmer for five minutes.

6. Add coconut milk and simmer for further five minutes.

7. Add salt to taste.

# Coconut Sambol

## (EASY)

### INGREDIENTS

- **Dry red chillies (roasted);** 6
- **\*Scraped coconut;** 1 cup
- **Onion (finely chopped;** 3 tbsp.
- **Lime juice;** 1 tsp
- **Salt;** to taste

\*Desiccated coconut can be used instead by microwaving it with little milk for 50 seconds.

## METHOD

1. Use a grinder or mortar to grind well the red chillies with salt.
2. Add onions, coconut and lime juice and blend at low speed.

# *Date Chutney*

## (EASY)

| INGREDIENTS |
|---|

- **Dates (ground);** 200 grams
- **Chilli powder;** 1 tbsp.
- **Ginger (ground);** 1 tbsp.
- **Garlic (ground);** 1 tbsp.
- **Sugar;** 200 grams
- **Vinegar;** 1/4 bottle
- **Salt;** to taste

## METHOD

1.  Mix all ingredients and boil well.  Bottle when cool.

# Date & Tomato Chutney

## (EASY)

| INGREDIENTS |
| --- |

- **Dates (ground);** 100 grams
- **Tomatoes;** 150 grams
- **Sugar;** 200 grams
- **Salt;** optional
- **Vinegar;** 1 cup
- Make a paste by grinding the following:
- **Ginger;** 2 tbsp.
- **Garlic;** 4 cloves
- **Mustard seeds;** 1 tsp
- **Dry chillies;** 10 -12
- **Vinegar;** 1 tbsp.

# METHOD

1. Scald the tomatoes by pouring hot water and remove the skin. Cut into small pieces.

2. Boil the tomatoes and dates in vinegar until the dates are soft.

3. Add the sugar, the paste, and salt and boil until a good consistency for chutney is reached.

4. Test the consistency by taking cold water in a saucer and putting a drop of the chutney. If it does not disintegrate the right consistency is reached.

5. Cool and bottle

# Fried Aubergine Pickle

## (MODERATE)

| INGREDIENTS |
| --- |

- **Aubergine (large);** 1
- **Oil (for frying);** as desired
- **Ginger (fresh root, small piece, crushed);** 1
- **Green chilli (finely chopped);** 1
- **Onion (red, medium, finely chopped);** 1/2
- **Turmeric powder (ground);** 1/2 tsp
- **Chilli powder;** 1/2 tsp
- **Vinegar;** 1/2 tsp
- **Lemon juice;** 1 tbsp.
- **Salt;** to taste
- **Black pepper;** to taste

# METHOD

1. Wash the eggplant and cut into thin strips.

2. Heat the oil in a pan

3. When the oil is hot, deep fry the eggplant in small batches until golden brown. Drain excess oil and set aside.

4. Add turmeric and chilli powder and toss well.

5. Add crushed ginger and the remaining ingredients to the eggplant

6. Add salt and black pepper to taste.

7. Mix thoroughly and serve.

# Hot and Sweet Seeni Sambol

## (EASY)

<table>
<tr><th colspan="2">INGREDIENTS</th></tr>
</table>

- **Onions (thinly sliced);** 3 (big)
- **Oil;** 3 tbsp.
- **Chilli powder;** 1 tsp
- **Tamarind paste;** 1 tbsp.
- **Water;** 4 tbsp.
- **Sugar;** 1 tbsp.
- **Salt;** 1 tsp

## METHOD

1. Heat the oil in a pan and fry the onions till they turn golden in colour.

2. Keep stirring frequently to stop burning.

3. Then add chilli powder and mix.

4. Next add the tamarind paste and water.

5. Cook till the mixture thickens.

6. Add the sugar and salt and mix well.

7. Enjoy with fresh bread.

# Vallarai Sambol

## (EASY)

| INGREDIENTS |
|---|
| • **Vallarai leaves (finely sliced);** 1 cup (Vallarai Keerai is called Brahmi leaves in English) |
| • **Red onion (finely sliced);** 1 |
| • **Coconut (fresh, scraped);** 2-3 tbsp. |
| • **Green chillies;** 2-3 |
| • **Pepper;** 1/4 tsp |
| • **Salt;** to taste |

## METHOD

1. Mix all ingredients well, bruising leaves with fingers to release aroma and taste.

# Jasmine's
# TAMIL
# KITCHEN

## SALADS

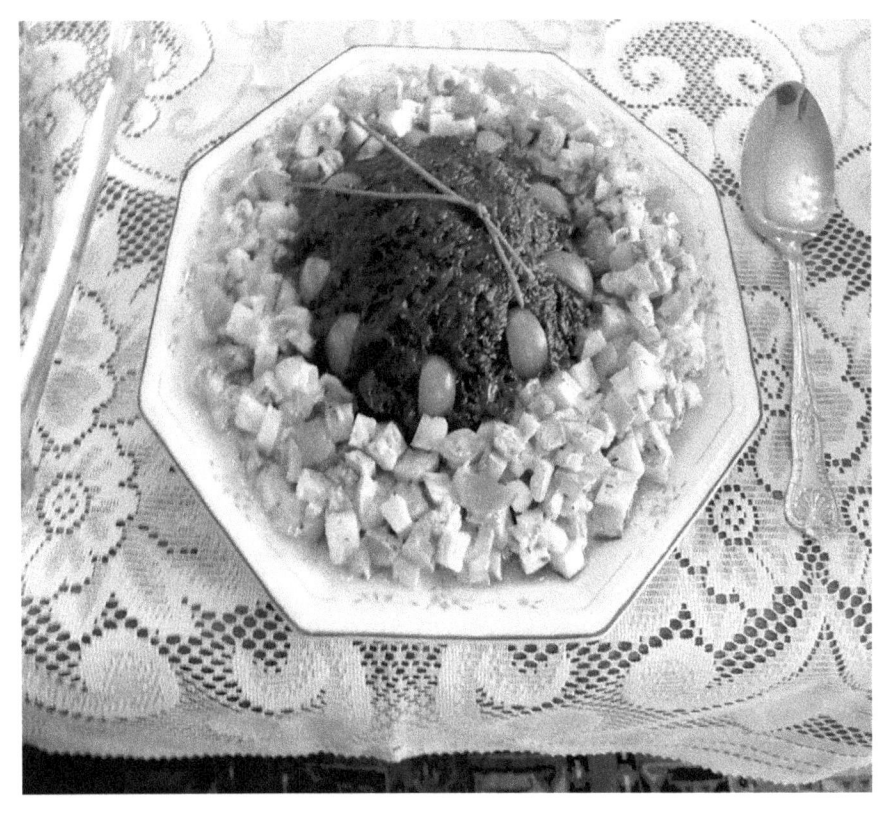

# Aubergine & Potato Salad

## (EASY)

| INGREDIENTS |
| --- |

- **Aubergine;** 1
- **Potato;** 1
- **Red onion (chopped);** ½
  **or spring onion;** 1
- **Coriander leaves (chopped);** 1 tbsp.
- **Yoghurt;** 250 grams
- **Lemon juice;** to taste
- **Salt;** to taste

## METHOD

1. Cut the aubergine into small squares.
2. Deep fry and let the oil drain for few hours.
3. Boil the potato and let it cool.

4.	Cut the potato into small squares.

5.	Finely chop the red onion or the spring onion.

6.	Mix the aubergine and potato with the rest of the ingredients.

7.	Serve and enjoy.

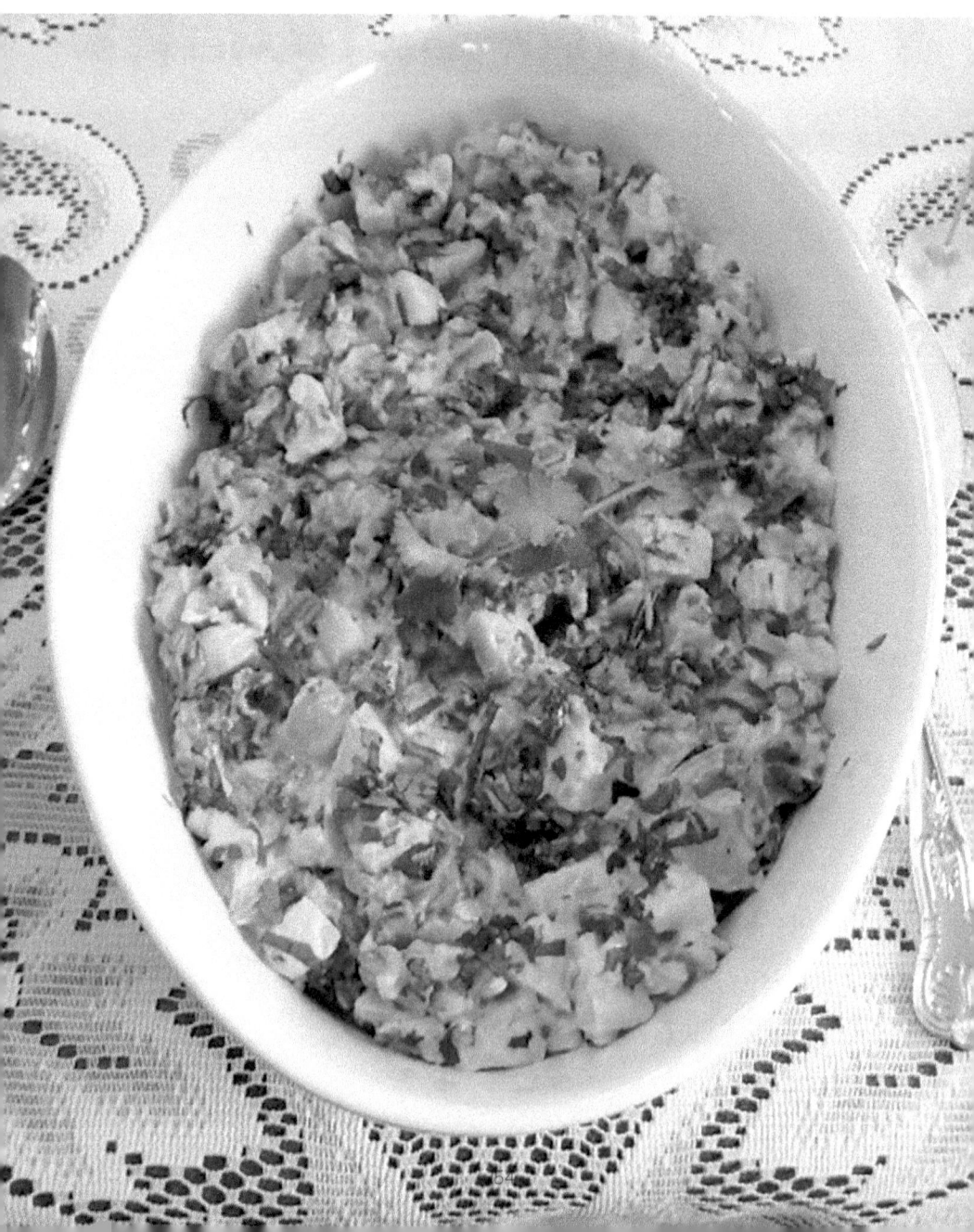

# Beetroot Salad

## (EASY)

| INGREDIENTS |
|---|

- **Beetroot;** 1
- **Green chillies;** 2
- **Onion (chopped);** 2 tbsp.
- **Lime juice;** 1 tsp
- **Yoghurt or cream;** 2 tbsp.
- **Salt;** to taste

## METHOD

1. Wash and cook beetroot in the oven OR boil the beetroot until tender.
2. Peel skin and grate or cut into very small pieces.
3. Mix in with the rest of the ingredients and serve.

# Cucumber & Tomato Salad

## (EASY)

| INGREDIENTS |
| --- |

- **Cucumber (chopped);** 1 cup
- **Tomato (chopped);** 1 ½ cup
- **Red onion (chopped);** 1 cup
- **Green chillies;** 2 or 3
- **Lime juice;** 1 tsp
- **Yoghurt (Greek);** 2 tbsp.
- **Pepper;** ¼ tsp
- **Salt;** to taste

## METHOD

1.  Mix in all the ingredients.

# Mixed Vegetable Salad

## (EASY)

<table>
<tr><th>INGREDIENTS</th></tr>
</table>

- **Cucumber;** 1
- **Tomatoes;** 2
- **Onion;** 1
- **Carrot;** 1
- **Green Apple;** 1
- **Lime juice;** 1/2 a lime
- **Pepper powder;** 1 tsp
- **Green chilies (cut into pieces);** 3
- **Salt;** to taste

## METHOD

1. Cut all vegetables and mix them with lime juice, pepper and salt.

2. Spread the cut pieces of green chilies on top of the vegetables and serve

80

# Yoghurt Salad

## (EASY)

| INGREDIENTS |
| --- |
| • **Yoghurt (heaped tea spoons)**; 2 -3 |
| • **Carrot (grated)**; 2 - 3 tbsp. (or cucumber; 1) |
| • **Onion (diced)**; 1 tbsp. |
| • **Green Chilli (cut into pieces)**; 1 |
| • **Coriander leaves (chopped)**; 1 tbsp. |
| • **Lemon juice;** to taste |
| • **Salt;** to taste |

## NOTE:

Grated carrot may be replaced by Cucumber. Cucumber needs to be skinned, de-seeded and diced or grated.

You may also use mint leaves instead of coriander leaves.

## METHOD

1.  Mix all ingredients in a bowl and the salad is ready to eat.

158

# *Jasmine's*
# TAMIL
# KITCHEN

## SOUPS

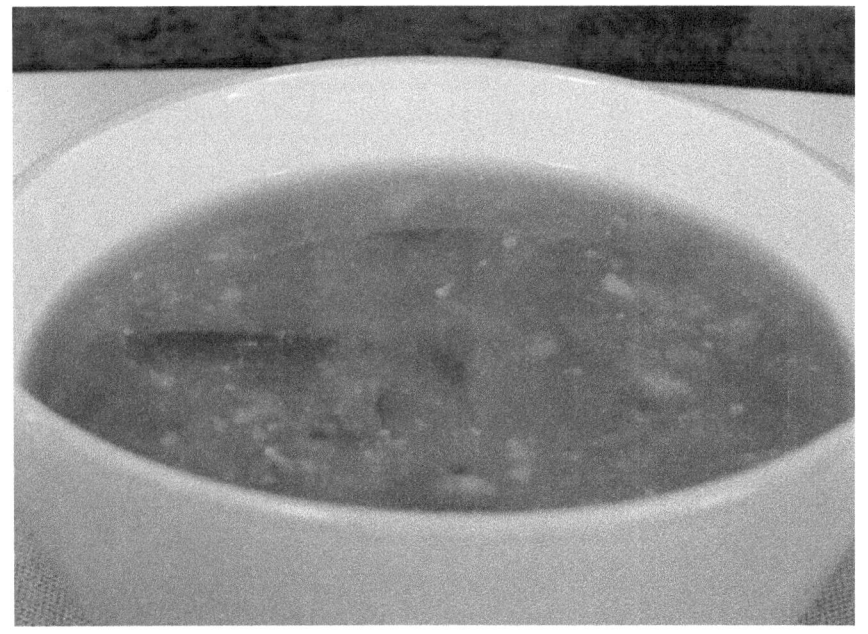

# 81

# Carrot and Coriander Soup

## (EASY)

| INGREDIENTS |
| --- |

- **Carrots (peeled & chopped);** 500 grams
- **Oil;** 1 tbsp.
- **Onion (chopped);** 1
- **Water;** 5 cups
- **Vegetable or chicken stock;** 1 cube
- **Coriander leaves (chopped);** a handful
- **Salt;** to taste
- **Single cream;** 1 or 2 tbsp.(optional)

## METHOD

1. Heat the oil in a pan, add the onions and fry.

2. Add carrots, water and stock cube. Stir and bring to boil.

3. Reduce the heat and cook until the carrots are tender.

4.  Turn off heat. Add the coriander leaves, mash it or blend in a food processor.

5.  Serve in a bowl, stir in the cream, and sprinkle a little coriander leaves.

# Dhal Rasam

## (CHALLENGING)

### INGREDIENTS

- **Toor dhal;** 1/4 cup
- **Dry chilli;** 1
- **Garlic;** 3 cloves
- **Water;** 2 cups
- **Turmeric powder;** 1/2 tsp
- **Coriander;** 1 tsp
- **Pepper;** 1/2 tsp
- **Cumin seeds;** 1/2 tsp
- **Tamarind juice;** 2 tbsp.
- **Tomato;** 1
- **Salt;** to taste

### METHOD

1. Wash and soak the dhal in 1 cup of water for about an hour.

2. Place the soaked dhal including the water in a pan and boil until the dhal is soft.

3.    Dry roast the chillies, coriander, pepper and cumin. Grind into fine powder.

4.    Boil the tamarind juice, crushed garlic, tomatoes and the ground powder in 1 cup of water for 5 minutes.  Add the dhal and simmer for 5 minutes.

5.    In a separate frying pan temper the following (additional ingredients) in 2 tsp hot oil for two minutes.

      **Onion (sliced)** 1; **Curry leaves;** 1 sprig and
      **Dry chilli (chopped);** 1

6.    Add cumin (1/2 tsp) and mustard (1/2 tsp) and temper for a further minute.

7.    Remove from the fire and add the tempered ingredients to the dhal water. Mix well.

# Jaffna Kool

## (CHALLENGING)

# 83

### INGREDIENTS

- **Fish;** 150 grams
- **Cuttlefish;** 150 grams
- **Prawns (small);** 150 grams
- **Crab;** 150 grams
- **Beans (long);** 100 grams
- **Cassava;** 100 grams
- **Jackfruit seeds (optional);** 100 grams
- **Murunga leaves;** 100 grams
- **Rice;** 3 tbsp.
- **Palmyrah root flour;** 1/2 cup
- **Dry chilli (cut into small pieces);** 10
- **Tamarind paste;** 1/2 tsp
- **Turmeric powder;** 1/2 tsp
- **Water;** 8 cups
- **Salt;** to taste

# METHOD

**Stage 1:**

1. Clean and wash the fish and the cuttlefish. Cut the fish into large pieces and the cuttlefish into small pieces.

2. Remove the shells from the prawns.

3. Wash and quarter the crabs

4. Break the beans into 3 cm pieces

5. Peel and dice the cassava.

6. Wash and chop the murunga leaves

7. Cut the Jack seeds into halves and then peel off the skin.

8. Soak the palmyrah root flour in water for ten minutes and then strain the water off.

9. Dissolve the tamarind in a cup of water for ten minutes and then strain and retain the water.

**Stage 2**

1. Half fill a large pan with water and bring to boil.

2. Add, rice, beans, cassava, jack seeds and salt and cook.

3. Half way through cooking add the fish, cuttle fish, prawns and crabs.

4. Mix in the Murunga leaves.

5. In a separate bowl mix the palmyrah root flour, tamarind solution, chilli powder and turmeric to get a thick paste.

6. Add this paste to the boiling mixture, and simmer until it thickens. Remove from the fire as soon as preferred consistency is reached.

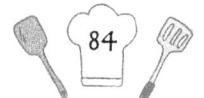

# Sour Vegetable Soup

## (CHALLENGING)

| INGREDIENTS |
| --- |

- Mixed vegetables (e.g. Eggplant, Long beans etc.); 1 ¼ cup
- Red raw rice; 1 ¼ cup
- Green chillies; 2
- Turmeric; 1/4 tsp
- Chilli powder; 1 tsp
- Tamarind juice; 2 tbsp.
- Coconut milk; 3 tbsp.
- Murunga leaves; 2 sprigs
- Water; 3 -4 cups
- A paste obtained by grinding the following:
- 1 tsp coriander, ½ tsp pepper, ½ tsp cumin seed and 10 garlic cloves.
- Salt; to taste

# METHOD

1. Boil the red raw rice in 2 cups of water.

2. When the rice is half cooked add the vegetables, green chillies and turmeric powder.

3. Add one more cup of water and continue to cook till the vegetables are fully cooked.

4. Now add salt, the paste and a further ½ cup of water.

5. Add the tamarind, coconut milk, murunga leaves and allow to simmer for a minute.

6. Serve hot.

# Vegetable Soup

## (EASY)

| INGREDIENTS |
|---|
| • **Carrots;** 100 grams |
| • **Beans;** 100 grams |
| • **Potato;** 100 grams |
| • **Cauliflower;** 100 grams |
| • **Water;** 1 ½ - 2 cups |
| • **Pepper powder;** 1 tsp |
| • **Salt;** to taste |

## METHOD

1. Steam the vegetables and allow to cool.

2. Mash the vegetables and add water, pepper powder, salt and boil.

3. Enjoy the soup when it has cooled to the required temperature.

# *Jasmine's*
# TAMIL
# KITCHEN

### SNACKS

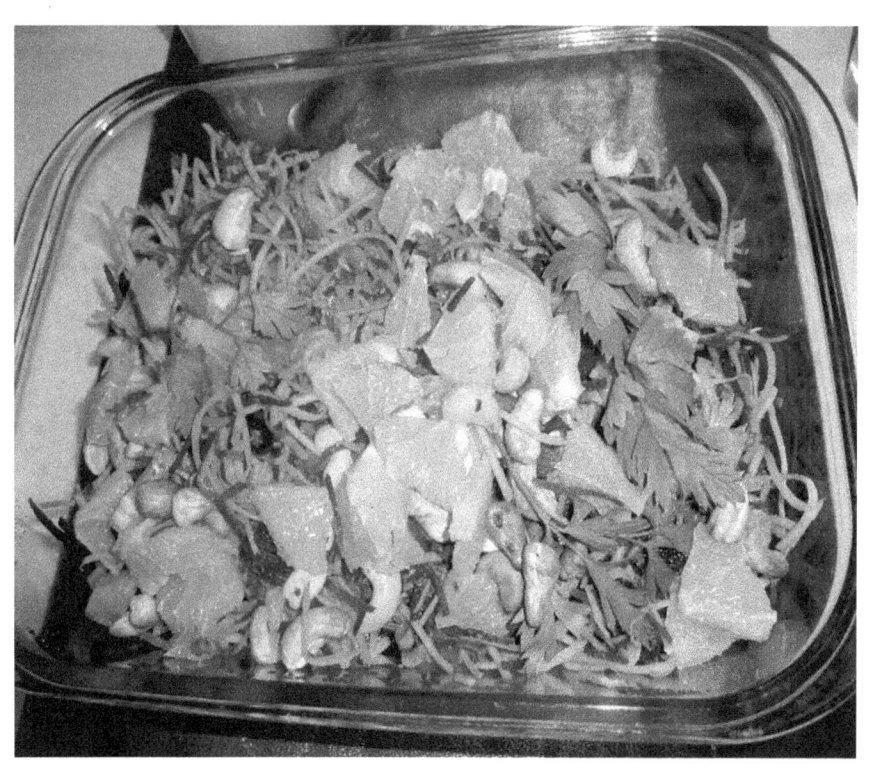

# Chick Pea Stir-fry

## (EASY)

### INGREDIENTS

- **Chick pea (washed and drained);** 1 tin
- **Oil;** 2 tbsp.
- **Onion (medium, chopped);** 1
- **Dry red chillies (cut into small pieces);** 2
- **Curry leaves;** 1 sprig
- **Mustard seeds;** 1/2 tsp
- **Fennel seeds;** 1/2 tsp
- **Salt;** to taste
- **Coconut (small cut pieces);** 2 tbsp.

# METHOD

1.  Fry the onion, red chillies and curry leaves in oil.

2.  Add mustard seeds and fennel seeds and continue to fry.

3.  To this add chick peas and salt and fry till chick peas get warmed up.

4.  Add the coconut cut pieces.

# *Green Mung Balls*

## (EASY)

| INGREDIENTS |
|---|
| • **Mung dhal (half roasted)** - 100g |
| • **Scraped coconut**; 50 grams |
| • **Sugar (or Scraped Jaggery)**; 2-3 tbsp. |
| • **Water:** 1 -2 cups |
| • **Salt:** to taste |

## METHOD

1. Boil the mung dhal in water with little salt till well cooked. When the dhal is soft drain the water.

2. Put dhal, scraped coconut and sugar or jaggery into a grinder (or a mortar) and grind.

3. Make Mung balls of the desired size.

# Kolukattai

## (CHALLENGING)

| INGREDIENTS |
| --- |

- **Red rice Flour**; 1 cup
- **Plain flour, steamed**; 1/4 cup
- **Salt**; 1/4 tbsp.
- **Hot Water**; 1/2 – 1 cup
- **Green gram, roasted**; 1/2 cup
- **Jaggery (or sugar)**; 1/4 cup
- **Coconut (fresh or desiccated)**; 1/2 cup
- **Cardamom powder**; to taste

## METHOD

1. Mix the red rice flour, plain flour and salt. Pour enough hot water to form a soft pliable (not watery) dough. Keep aside.

2. Prepare the filling for the kolukattai by mixing the roasted green gram made into granules (ie boiled in 1 ½ cups of water with a pinch of salt until the water is absorbed) with coconut, jaggery and cardamom powder.

3. Roll out the dough between two sheets of cling wrap

4. Cut the rolled out dough into circles.

5. Fill the cut out circles with 1 ½ tsp of the filling.

6. Fold the circle to form a semi-circle and press the edges with fingertips to seal the ends (A fork can be used instead)

7. Arrange the kolukattai in a steamer and steam for 10 minutes.

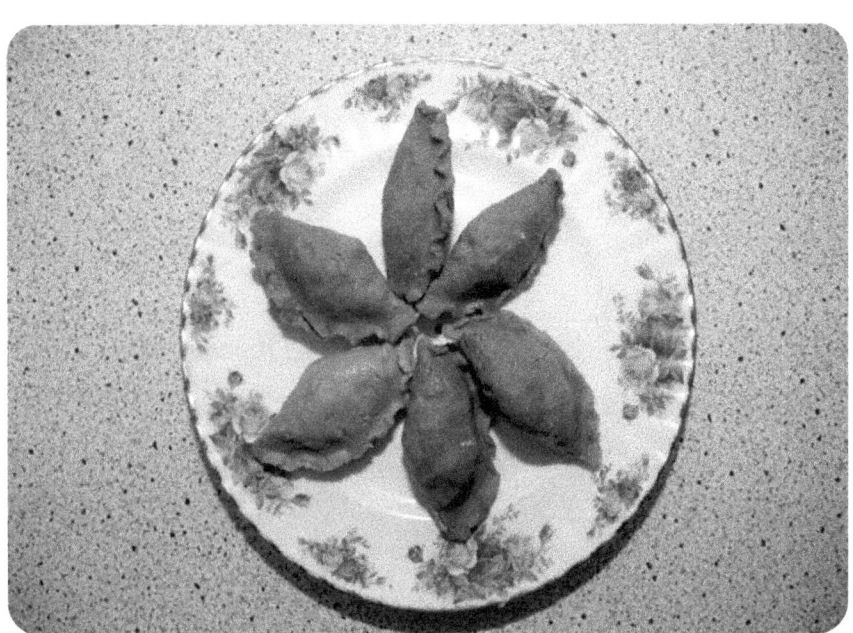

# Meat Cutlet

## (CHALLENGING)

| INGREDIENTS |
| --- |

- **Minced beef (or lamb);** 250 grams
- **Onion –** 1
- **Oil;** 2-3 tbsp.
- **Potatoes;** 1- 2
- **Green chillies (split);** 2
- **Curry leaves;** 1 sprig
- **Garlic (crushed);** 1 tsp
- **Ginger (crushed);** 1 tsp
- **Pepper (powder);** 1/2 tsp
- **Chilli powder;** 1 tbsp.
- **Curry powder;** 1 tsp
- **Bread crumbs;** (as required)
- **Lemon (or lime);** 1/4
- **Egg;** 1
- **Cardamom/cloves (optional); 2** or 3
- **Water;** as necessary
- **Salt; to** taste

# METHOD

1. Cut the potato into pieces and boil for 20 minutes or till able to mash easily.

2. Temper the onion, curry leaves, chillies, garlic and ginger in 2-3 tbsp. of oil.

3. Add the minced meat, mash potatoes, salt, lemon/lime, pepper, chilli powder and curry powder and stir.

**Batter:**

4. Make the batter as follows:

5. Mix 1/4 cup of plain white flour, 1 beaten egg, salt, pepper and water(as necessary) to get the right consistency.(i.e. not too thick)

6. Make balls out of the meat mixture.

7. Dip each meat ball in the batter and then in the bread crumbs and fry in oil till they turn dark brown.

# *Patties*

## (CHALLENGING)

### INGREDIENTS FOR THE FILLING

- **Meat;** 100 grams
- **Potatoes;** 50 grams
- **Oil;** 1 tbsp.
- **Mustard seeds;** 1/4 tsp
- **Cumin seeds;** 1/4 tsp
- **Onion (medium, sliced);** 1
- **Green chilli (sliced);** 1
- **Ginger & garlic paste;** 1 tsp
- **Tomato (chopped);** 1
- **Curry powder;** 2 tsp
- **Turmeric;** a pinch

### INGREDIENTS FOR THE PASTRY

- **Flour (plain);** 1 cup
- **Butter;** 2 tsp
- **Salt;** to taste
- **Cold water**
- **Oil for frying**

# METHOD

**Method for making the filling**

1. Boil the meat and potatoes and cut both into small pieces. Set aside.

2. Heat the oil in a pan and add mustard seeds, cumin seeds, onion, green chilli and ginger-garlic paste and sauté.

3. Add chopped tomato, curry powder and turmeric and continue to sauté. Finally add the meat and potatoes and mix well.

**Method for making the pastry:**

1. Mix flour, salt and butter into a crumble. Then add cold water to make a thick dough. Wrap this dough in a cling foil and refrigerate for half an hour.

**Method for making the Patties**

1. Roll the dough to ¼ cm thick and cut circular pieces of 7cm diameter each.

2. Place a table spoon of filling on half of each circular piece. To make the dough stick well, wet the rim with water.

3. Fold the other half on top of the filling mixture and press the rims together with a fork.

4. Place all the patties on a floured plate.

5. Fry the patties in hot oil till they turn to a golden colour.

# Sweet Corn Preparation

## (EASY)

| INGREDIENTS |
| --- |
| • **Sweet corn;** 1 or 2 pieces<br>• **Butter;** 1/2 tsp<br>• **Salt;** to taste |

### METHOD

1. Place the corn in a microwave safe container.

2. Sprinkle a handful of water.

3. If the container has no airtight cover, cover tightly with cling wrap.

4. Place in microwave and cook on high for 3 minutes.

5. Apply the butter and let it melt and cover the corn.

6. Return to the microwave and cook on low for 2 minutes.

7. Transfer to a plate and sprinkle salt to taste.

# *Jasmine's*
# TAMIL
# KITCHEN

## SWEETS & DESSERTS

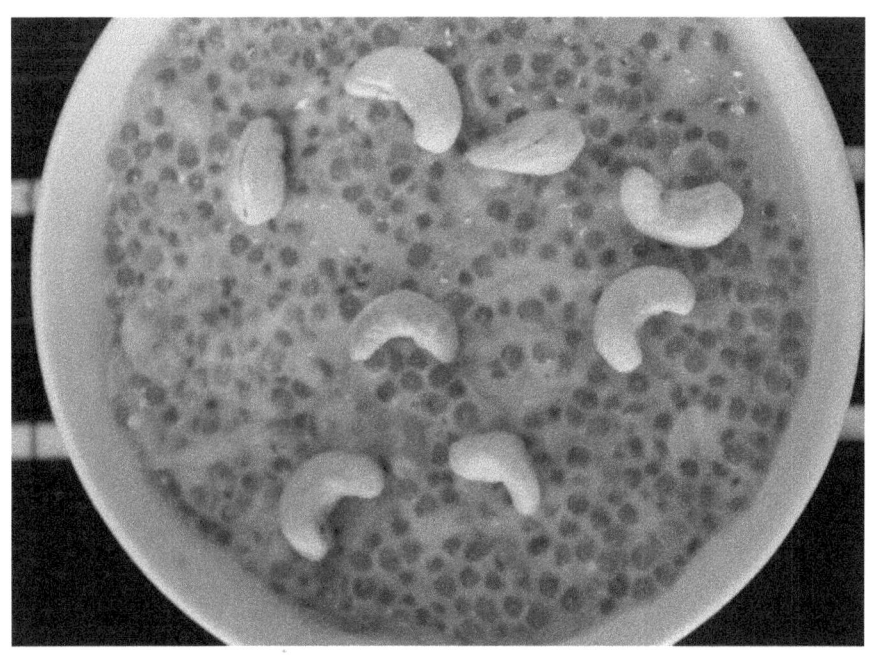

# Apple and Almond Cake

## (EASY)

- **Apple (cored and chopped);** 1/4 kg
- **Caster sugar;** 2 tbsp.
- **Self-rising flour;** 2 tbsp.
- **Margarine;** 1 tbsp.
- **Egg;** 1
- **Flaked almonds;** 1/2 tbsp.

## METHOD

1. Obtain a cake mixt by mixing together the Margarine, sugar, egg and flour one at a time in the order.

2. In a clear Pyrex dish or bowl spread a little of the chopped apple cover with a layer of cake mix then layers of chopped apples and cake mix, finally with the cake mixture on top.

3. Sprinkle with flaked Almond and Bake for 1 ½ hours.

# Bread Pudding

## (EASY)

| INGREDIENTS |
|---|

- **Bread (cut into cubes);** 3 slices
- **Milk;** 1 cup
- **Butter;** 2 tbsp.
- **Thick cream;** 1 cup
- **Eggs (large);** 2
- **Sugar (or grated jaggery);** 1/2 cup
- **Salt; a** pinch
- **Vanilla;** 1 tsp
- **Raisins; 1**/2 cup
- **Cashew nuts (chopped);** 2 tbsp.
- **Cinnamon powder; a** pinch
- **Lemon peel (grated);** 1 lemon
- **Water (boiled);** as required

# METHOD

1. Butter the baking dish and set aside.

2. Put bread cubes in a large bowl

3. Heat the milk and cream in a pan. Set aside.

4. Whisk egg, sugar, salt, vanilla, cinnamon and grated lemon peel in a medium bowl.

5. Transfer the milk and cream into the egg mixture and pour this over bread and combine the mixture; let it stand for half an hour.

6. Add raisins and cashew nuts to the bread mixture and pour the mixture into the buttered dish.

7. Set dish in a roasting pan with boiling water in the pan half way up the sides of dish.

8. Pre heat oven to 180 degrees Celsius; bake until golden brown & cool dish for 10 to 20 minutes.

# Carrot Halwa

## (EASY)

| INGREDIENTS |
|---|

- **Carrot;** 250 grams
- **Sugar;** 250 grams
- **Milk;** 1 cup
- **Butter;** 100 grams
- **Cardamoms;** 4
- **Cashew nuts;** 15

## METHOD

1. Wash the carrots, peel the skin and grate.
2. Boil the carrots in milk for 30 mins.
3. Add sugar and when it is caramelised add butter.
4. Add cashew nuts and cardamoms.
5. Pour the mixture into a buttered dish.
6. Cut into pieces and serve.

# Eggless Butter Cake

## (EASY)

### INGREDIENTS

- **Condensed milk;** 1 cup
- **Water;** 3/4 cup
- **Butter;** 250 grams
- **Sugar;** 3 tbsp.
- **Flour (plain);** 250 grams
- **Baking powder;** 2 tsp
- **Honey;** 2 tbsp.
- **Desiccated coconut;** 1/2 cup
- **Juice of half a lime and half an orange.**

# METHOD

1. Mix milk, flour and water.

2. In a separate bowl beat sugar and butter; add to the milk flour mixture.

3. Add juices, honey, coconut and baking powder.

4. Transfer the mixture to a greased and line prepared tin.

5. Bake in an oven at 160 degrees Celsius for 40 minutes

# Green Gram Sweet

## (EASY)

### INGREDIENTS

- **Green gram flour (roasted);** 150 grams
- **Desiccated coconut**; 100grams
- **Sugar;** 250 grams
- **Pepper (powdered);** 1/2 tsp
- **Cumin seeds;** 1/2 tsp
- **Plain flour;** 100 grams
- **White rice flour;** 100 grams
- **Oil for frying;** as required
- **Hot water;** little
- **Salt;** to taste

# METHOD

1.  Roast the desiccated coconut until golden brown and grind.

2.  Grind the sugar.

3.  Mix the first five ingredients together adding a little hot water. (Mix as if preparing for pittu).

4.  Make small balls.

5.  Make batter with plain flour, white rice flour and salt.

6.  Dip the balls in the batter and fry in the oil.

# Kesari

## (CHALLENGING)

| INGREDIENTS |
| --- |

- **Semolina (roasted);** 1/2 cup
- **Sugar;** 3/4 cup
- **Butter;** 3 tbsp.
- **Ghee;** 3 tbsp.
- **Cashew nuts (cut into pieces);** 10
- **Raisins;** 1 tbsp.
- **Kesari powder;** a pinch
- **Cardamom powder;** 1/2 tsp
- **Water;** 1 ¼ cups

## METHOD

1. Keep a buttered tray ready.

2. Warm the water and stir in sugar until it dissolves. Keep this sugar syrup aside.

3. Melt the butter in a pan on low heat. Roast the cashew nuts in it and when they turn to a golden colour add the raisins; remove from the pan and keep aside.

4. To the remaining butter in the pan add the semolina and roast till it turns to a golden colour with a nice aroma.

5. Add the sugar syrup and kesari powder and mix well. Increase the heat and cook till the water and sugar syrup are absorbed.

6. Reduce the heat, add ghee and continue to cook.

7. Add cashew nuts, raisins and cardamom powder and mix well.

8. Transfer this mixture on to the buttered tray and flatten with the back of the spoon. Let it cool.

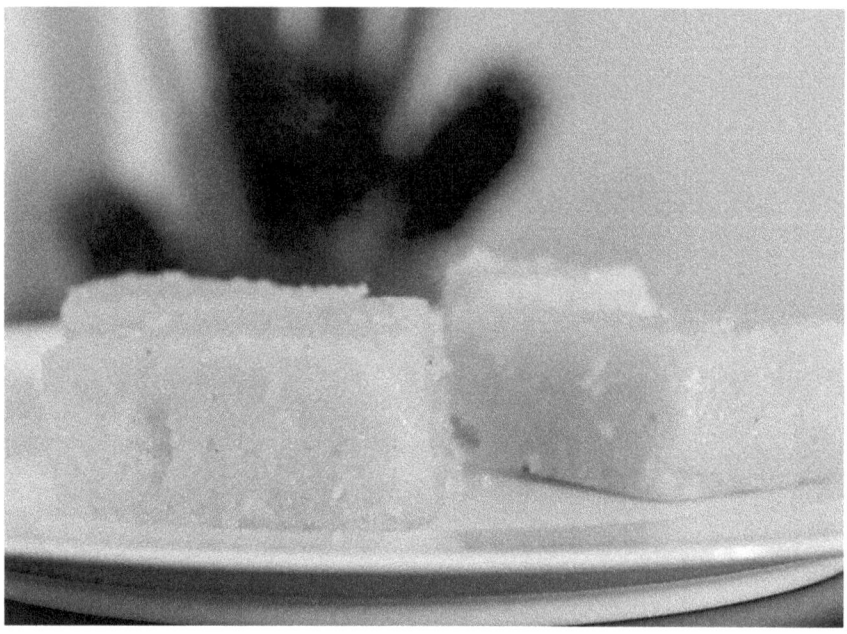

# King Yam Pudding (Rasavalli)

## [EASY]

- **King Yam;** 200 grams
- **Sugar; 50 grams**
- **Coconut milk;** 1 cup
- **Water;** (enough to cover the yam)
- **Salt;** 1/4 tsp.

## METHOD

1. Peel the king yam, cut into slices and wash thoroughly.

2. Boil the yam in water and salt until soft.

3. Add sugar and mash the yam.

4.  Add the coconut milk and cook the mixture until it thickens.

5.  Take off fire and cool.

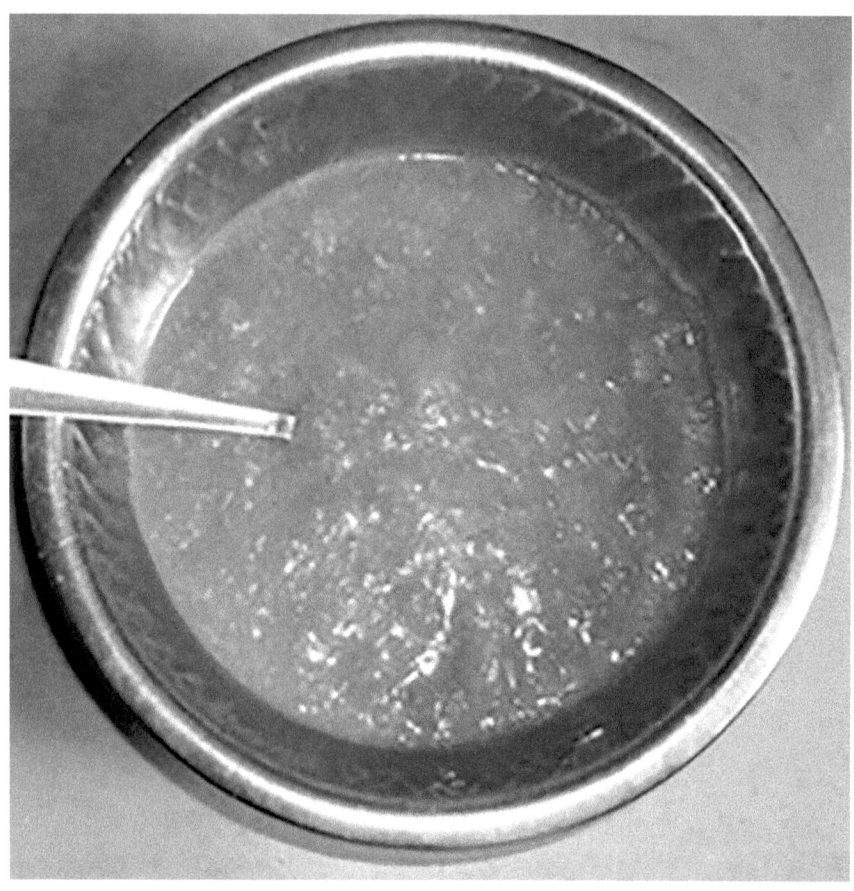

# King Yam Pudding

## (CHALLENGING)

| INGREDIENTS |
|---|

- **King Yam;** 250 grams
- **Coconut milk (thick);** 1/2 cup (first milk, thick)
- **Coconut milk (thin);** 1 cup (second milk, thin)
- **Sugar;** 50 grams
- **Salt;** to taste

## METHOD

1. Peel and cut the yam into slices.

2. Wash well and cook in a pan with the thin second coconut milk until soft.

3. Remove from the fire and mash the yam.

4.  Add the thick first coconut milk and sugar and cook until the sugar has dissolved and the milk has boiled. Add salt to taste.

5.  Serve hot or cold. [Note that once cold, the mixture will become a smooth firm paste]

# Laddu

## (EASY)

| INGREDIENTS |
|---|

- **Semolina;** 100 grams
- **Butter;** 2 tbsp.
- **Sugar;** 50 grams
- **Cashew nuts (chopped);** 10
- **Sultanas;** 1 tbsp.
- **Milk;** 1/4 – 1/2 cup
- **Cardamom powder;** 1 tsp

## METHOD

1. Melt the butter.
2. Fry chopped cashew nuts and sultanas. Keep aside.
3. Roast the semolina till it is slightly brown.
4. Add the sugar to semolina and continue roasting till the sugar starts to melt and the mixture begins to form tiny lumps.
5. Add the cardamom powder, cashew nuts and sultanas.
6. Add the milk little at a time and mix well.
7. Make balls from the semolina mixture while hot.

# Payasam

## (EASY)

| INGREDIENTS |
| --- |

- **Sago;** 50 grams
- **Butter;** 1 tbsp.
- **Coconut milk;** 2 cups
- **Cashew (chopped);** 1 tbs.
- **Raisins;** 1 tbsp.
- **Sugar;** 2 tsp
- **Water;** 1 cup
- **Vermicelli;** 2 tbsp.
- **Cardamom powder;** 1/4 tsp

## METHOD

1. Fry cashew and raisins in butter (keep aside).

2. Roast sago in butter till golden in colour, add water and cook until transparent.

3. Add vermicelli and cook till the mixture thickens.

4. Mix in coconut milk, sugar and cardamom powder and cook for 3 minutes longer.

5. Finally add cashew and raisins.

6. Serve hot or cold.

# Pine Apple Upside-down Cake

## (CHALLENGING)

| INGREDIENTS |
| --- |

- **Butter**; 125 grams
- **Caster sugar**; 3/4 cup
- **Eggs; 2**
- **Self-rising flour**; 250 grams
- **Milk**; 1/4 cup
- **Pine apple syrup**; 1/4 cup
- **Ingredients (for topping)**
- **Butter**; 60 grams
- **Brown sugar**; 1/2 cup
- **Pine apple slices**; 1 can
  ((about 450 grams)
- **Cherries**; 6-8

# METHOD

1. Mix butter and sugar. Add eggs one by one beating them until light and fluffy

2. Add in flour and milk and pineapple syrup and beat lightly until smooth. Leave it aside.

3. Blend soft butter with brown sugar and spread it over the base of a greased deep cake tin. Arrange the pineapple slices and cherries over the brown sugar mixture.

4. Spread the cake mixture evenly over the pineapple slices and bake for one hour at 180 degrees Celsius.

5. Wait for a few minutes and transfer the cake onto a serving plate. Enjoy with custard/cream.

# 103

# Sago Pudding

## (EASY)

| INGREDIENTS |
|---|
| • **Sago;** 100 grams |
| • **Milk (Coconut milk preferred);** 2 cups |
| • **Ghee or Butter;** 1 tbsp. |
| • **Cashew nuts (chopped);** 2 tbsp. |
| • **Water;** 1 cup |
| • **Vermicelli;** 5 grams |
| • **Sugar;** 100 grams |
| • **Cardamom; 5** (powdered) |
| • **Raisins;** 1 tbsp. |

## METHOD

1. Roast the sago in ghee or butter to a golden colour.

2. Fry the cashew nuts and raisins separately in ghee.

3. Cook the sago in water until it is transparent.

4. Add the vermicelli and milk to sago and cook until the mixture thickens slightly.

5. Mix in the sugar and the cardamom powder and cook for 5 minutes

6. Mix the cashew nuts and raisins with the sago mixture and serve hot or cold.

# 104

# Semolina Sweet

## (EASY)

| INGREDIENTS |
| --- |

- **Semolina;** 500 grams
- **Sugar;** 250 grams
- **Margarine;** 125 grams
- **Desiccated coconut;** 1 cup
- **Eggs;** 2
- **Cashew nuts;** 50 grams
- **Sultanas;** 50 grams
- **Nutmeg;** a few
- **Vanilla;** as required

## METHOD

1. Separate the eggs, beat the yolk of the egg and beat the egg white to froth.

2. Roast the Semolina mix in the sugar, margarine and mix.

3. Add the coconut, cashew nuts, sultanas and nutmeg and mix

4. Mix in the beaten egg York with vanilla.

5. Stir in the frothy egg white

6. Pour into a tray and bake in an oven.

# Wattalappam

## (CHALLENGING)

---

# 105

### INGREDIENTS

- **Condensed Milk;** 1 tin
- **Coconut Milk/Cream;** 1 tin
- **Jaggery or Palm Sugar;** 200gm
- **Brown Sugar;** 100gm
- **Eggs;** 5
- **Nutmeg;** 2 tsp
- **Powdered cardamom seeds (no husk);** 1/4 tsp
- **Cashew pieces (roasted);** optional  1/2 cup
- **Water;** 3 – 4 tbsp.

---

### METHOD

1. Pre-heat oven to 150 degrees.

2. Grate jaggery and heat it in water (or microwave on low).

3. Beat eggs with Jaggery and brown sugar and then add the nutmeg, cardamom, coconut milk and condensed milk.

4. Pour into a Pyrex dish and bake for 1 hour in the oven until set. (*Keep a bowl of water in the bottom shelf of the oven to get a steamed effect) - *optional

5. Add the cashew nuts three quarter way of baking the Wattalappam.

# RECIPE CONTRIBUTORS

I am fortunate to be surrounded by family and friends who are expert cooks; my gratitude goes out to all who helped compile the recipes in this book. Each recipe has the name of the contributor, and the list of the contributors below is in the alphabetical order of the Surnames together with their recipes.

**ALOYSIUS** Angelita, London, UK

**ASEERVATHAM** Jasmine (deceased) Favourites

**ASEERVATHAM** Shubu & Ratna. Sunshine Coast, Queensland, Australia

**Atputharajah** Delanie, North York, Ontario, Canada

**Christy** Jeanette, Brisbane, Qld., Australia

**Ferdinand** Joyce. Weely, Essex, UK

**Indraharan** Anusha, Melbourne, Australia

**Kandasamy** Radha. Melbourne, Australia

**Mahadevan** Christine, Ermington, NSW, Australia

**Manoharan** Sobana, Brisbane, Australia

**Santhiapillai** Elizabeth, North York, Canada

**Saravanabhava** Mala, Brisbane, Australia

**Sivananthan** Vasuki, Brisbane, Australia

**Soosaipillai** Regina, Glenwood, NSW, Australia

**Thevasagayam** Jasline, Wynum West, Australia

Fried Chicken.................................................................................P109

**Thomas** Dawn, Albany Creek, Queensland, Australia

Corned Beef Fry ...........................................................................P122
Yoghurt Salad.................................................................................P180
Sweet Corn Preparation...............................................................P205

**Thurairatnam** Caroline, Talopea, NSW, Australia

Lamb Curry ....................................................................................P124

**Vaheesan** Dhusyanthi

Drumstick Red Curry ..................................................................... P79
Wattalappam ...................................................................................
P234

**Veerasingam** Rajanie, O'malley, ACT, Australia

Cabbage and Carrot Stir Fry ........................................................ P71
Lentil Curry...................................................................................... P82
Spinach Curry.................................................................................. P96

www.ingramcontent.com/pod-product-compliance
Lightning Source LLC
Chambersburg PA
CBHW051142120626
46547CB00012B/907